110658418

The Deanna Protocol®

The Deanna Protocol®

Hope for ALS
and Other Neurological Conditions

Vincent M. Tedone, M.D.
Deanna Tedone-Gage
Chiara Tedone

paradies / inspire, llc
Tampa, Florida

© 2015 Winning the Fight, Inc.
All rights reserved. Published 2015.
Printed in the United States of America.

Published by paradies / inspire, llc
Tampa, Florida

No part of this book may be reproduced, stored in a retrieval system, or transmitted in any form or by any means, electronic, mechanical, photocopying, recording, or otherwise, without prior written permission of the publisher. Permissions may be sought directly by emailing the publisher at veronica@ paradiesinspire.com.

The Deanna Protocol® is a registered service mark of Winning the Fight, Inc.

ISBN: 978-1-941102-10-7 (hardcover)
ISBN: 978-1-941102-13-8 (paperback)
ISBN: 978-1-941102-12-1 (ePub ebook)

Book design by Jennifer Omner

Contents

PART TWO: A Call To Action

PART THREE: The Deanna Protocol®

Foreword

The Deanna Protocol: Hope for ALS is a story of a father's love, a daughter's courage and a family's resolve. Deanna and her father, Dr. Vince Tedone, want every patient suffering from ALS, who we refer to as PALS, to receive the nutritional support needed to fight this awful disease. The entire Tedone family has made this their cause. Countless hours have been invested in helping Winning the Fight, Inc., a charitable organization that they have established and lead to inform PALS about the Deanna Protocol®, the first effective treatment for ALS. They have supported research and raised money for other charities. They have never given up on Deanna, who has ALS, and continues her struggle to beat this disease.

Winning the Fight, Inc. helps PALS interested in implementing the Deanna Protocol® in their own lives through its website www.winningthefight.org. Through Winning the Fight, Inc., Dr. Tedone has sponsored research in an ALS mouse model, SOD1-G93A that confirms the benefits of the Deanna Protocol® observed in Deanna and reported by hundreds of PALS through the forums of www.winningthefight.org.

The Deanna Protocol is divided into three parts. *Part One* tells the story of the discovery of the Deanna Protocol® from the perspective of those most intimately involved in its discovery. In *Part Two*, the authors provide sound, scientific evidence that the Deanna Protocol® is an effective, metabolic therapy. *Part Three* provides advice in implementing the Deanna Protocol® as nutritional support for PALS or anyone suffering from a neurodegenerative disease.

As compelling as *Part One* of *The Deanna Protocol* is, there are many PALS who will not hear about the Deanna Protocol® or will hear only when it is too late to prevent irreversible damage. Also, there is so much more work that needs to be done. More documentation is necessary to convince neurologists to recommend the Deanna Protocol®. Scientists need a better understanding of how the Deanna Protocol® slows the progression of ALS. Winning the Fight, Inc. supports testing of a combination of the Deanna Protocol® with other therapies that can reverse the disease, if possible. This book is a call to action to PALS, clinicians and researchers.

The authors' hope is that more PALS will learn of the Deanna Protocol® by telling Deanna's story. Deanna is a private person, and it has been difficult for her to expose herself and her struggles with ALS in the pages of this book. The Tedone family is a private, normal family, which has been thrust into the center of this fight against ALS, because it is necessary to get the word out to PALS that the Deanna Protocol® works. PALS need to learn about the Deanna Protocol® as early as possible in the progression of this degenerative disease, before more irreversible damage is done.

Skepticism has a place, but healthy skepticism does not justify doing nothing. Nobody stands to gain anything from the success of the Deanna Protocol®, other than the benefit that PALS will receive. The Deanna Protocol® is not an expensive therapy. The authors are not selling anything, do not operate a clinic and are not seeking monetary gain. Indeed, the authors are working with supplement manufacturers to make the Deanna Protocol® even less expensive than it is today. Perhaps, this is part of the problem. There is no large pharmaceutical company, with a large marketing budget, to convince neurologists of the benefits of the Deanna Protocol®.

There is peer-reviewed research that the Deanna Protocol® slows or stops the progression of ALS, and it is not just anecdotal evidence.[1] Even the ability to slow the degeneration caused by this horrible disease provides an opportunity for clinicians to make a difference in the lives of their patients who might have ALS. To take advantage of this opportunity, every clinician who sees patients with neurodegenerative disease symptoms needs to know about the empirical evidence showing that PALS on the Deanna Protocol® live better, longer lives.

Waiting is not an option. The earlier that PALS start the Deanna Protocol® the better the results. The Deanna Protocol® gives PALS hope. Hope, not only of slowing this degenerative disease, but eventually, that researchers will

---

1   The Deanna Protocol® added to a standard diet significantly extended survival time of SOD1-G93A mice by 7.5% (p = 0.001), Ari C, Poff AM, Held HE, Landon CS, Goldhagen CR, et al., "Metabolic Therapy with Deanna Protocol Supplementation Delays Disease Progression and Extends Survival in Amyotrophic Lateral Sclerosis (ALS) Mouse Model," *PLoS ONE*, 9(7) (2014); see http://dx.plos.org/10.1371/journal.pone.0103526.

find an effective therapy for reversing the degeneration of motor neurons at the root of this dreadful disease. The authors and the researchers on Deanna's team are hot on the trail, but more resources are needed. More minds are needed. More research is needed.

Reviewing the history of over 1,000 PALS, worldwide, it takes about 2 years, on average, to eventually receive a diagnosis of ALS. The authors believe that it would be inexcusable to wait until there is anatomical evidence of diffuse extreme atrophy, before recommending the Deanna Protocol® to patients. The overwhelming evidence is that the Deanna Protocol® improves the quality of life of PALS with only modest inconvenience.

Deanna did not have time to wait for gene therapies to be developed. GDH and GAD, the enzymes that act on glutamate to produce AKG and GABA, were too unstable, were expensive to make and were not readily available. Dr. Tedone decided to do what could be done and to see if it produced any beneficial results. PALS do not have time to wait. It is past time that the Deanna Protocol® became part of the standard of care for PALS or any patient exhibiting symptoms of neurodegenerative diseases, in general, and motor neuron diseases, in particular.

All of the revenue from the sales of this book is directed to Winning the Fight, Inc., a charity that pays no salaries or benefits to any of its directors and executives. The publisher, Paradies / Inspire, has donated its contribution to this book. All of the charitable contributions to Winning the Fight, Inc. are directed to helping PALS and to conducting research to improve the therapies available to PALS. Winning the Fight, Inc. is planning to sponsor a clinical trial combining the Deanna Protocol® with other therapies that show promise in reversing the effects of ALS.

Giving patients information about the benefits of the Deanna Protocol® will do no harm, even if the patient does not have ALS. All of the supplements are inexpensive and readily available and are safe for human consumption in the amounts suggested in the Deanna Protocol®.

If you are a clinician, you need to recommend the Deanna Protocol® to your patients. It is safe and effective nutritional supplementation that supports motor neuron health. The evidence shows that ALS is a metabolic disorder that starves neurons of energy. The Deanna Protocol® is an alternative pathway for providing the neurons the energy needed to survive, when the ordinary energy cycle breaks down.

If you are a patient, you need to visit your caregiver and convince him or her that the Deanna Protocol® is worth trying. These chapters are a call to action for PALS, clinicians and researchers. Evaluate the evidence, dispassionately. Then, if you arrive at the same conclusions as the authors, join us. Help us find a cure. Win the fight against ALS, and win the fight against other neurodegenerative diseases.

If you would like to contribute to Winning the Fight, Inc. and make a real difference in the lives of PALS, you can go to their website: www.winningthefight.org.

Preface

The authors are in a life and death struggle against a terrible disease, Amyotrophic Lateral Sclerosis, which is referred to as ALS or Lou Gehrig's disease. If you or a loved one have been diagnosed with ALS, then you need to read this book. The Deanna Protocol® program was discovered by Dr. Tedone, Deanna's father, only after failing, again and again, with everything that he tried. The massage, non-exhausting exercise and core supplements are inexpensive and available without prescription from many suppliers. The program works for many ALS patients. It is not a cure; however, it provides a better quality of life and has been shown in ALS mice to extend life and improve motor skills. The rate of progression of ALS symptoms reported in ALSFRS scores, is markedly reduced in those adhering to the Deanna Protocol® program. There are few side effects reported, and those are manageable for most, if the program is phased in, gradually, over time.

The main stream pharmaceutical giants and neurologists have taken little notice or remain skeptical about any program targeting metabolic support of motor neurons. However, we are winning over some of the skeptics, when they see, first-hand, how much their own patients are benefiting from the Deanna Protocol® program.

An investigation at the University of South Florida has shown that SOD1-G93A mice live longer and better when on the core supplements of the Deanna Protocol® program. To our knowledge, the Deanna Protocol® program is the only program tested on these particular mice that has ever shown a statistically significant extension of life compared to controls. We were not surprised, because the program already showed effectiveness in Deanna and many other patients with ALS (PALS).

More surprising to us is the anecdotal evidence that the core supplements of the Deanna Protocol® program helps patients with other neurological conditions, such as Alzheimer's. An investigation of these other conditions is beyond our foundation's capability. We don't have sufficient assets to meet the needs for research into ALS. Much of the costs of the progress made to date have been borne by the Tedone's and a short list of donors to Winning the Fight, Inc., a foundation established by the Tedone family. If the foundation had more money, the research could progress much faster in ALS and other neurological conditions could be included, which have shown benefits to patients from taking the core supplements of the Deanna Protocol® program.

The authors are convinced that there is a common denominator among many neurological conditions that could, potentially, benefit from the Deanna Protocol® program or some program based on the core supplements of the Deanna Protocol® program. Possibly, Alzheimer's, Parkinson's, stroke, traumatic brain injury and other neurological conditions could all share a common pathway for neuron cell death, a lack of energy in the cells.

The authors believe that one of the supplements taken as part of the Deanna Protocol® program provides energy to distressed cells in which normal cellular metabolism has been disrupted. From research completed after the manuscript for this book was written, Dr. Tedone believes that many of these neurological conditions could benefit from a program tailored toward keeping more of the neurons from dying. This Preface and an Afterword have been added to the soft cover edition of this book. If you are interested in our efforts to discover a metabolic program for benefitting the health of patients with neurological conditions resulting in neuron cell death, then turn to the Afterword for a discussion on our evolving hypothesis.

Also, the Deanna Protocol® program continues to evolve over time as more research is conducted and more PALS report their results to us. Please go to www. winningthefight.org for the latest information and recommendations. If you register, report on your efforts to adhere to the Deanna Protocol® program, and provide us your ALSFRS scores, you will be helping us to battle ALS.

PART ONE

A Father's Love;
A Daughter's Courage;
A Family's Resolve

Chapter One

Deanna

In 2006, I married Don Gage, the love of my life. We first met in eighth grade in a romantic encounter typical for our age. I walked by him on the school bus. He looked right at me and snickered, "You have a big nose!" I rolled my eyes, as thirteen-year-old girls are likely to do, and fired back: "Well, at least *mine* doesn't look like a ski slope!" Walking away from him, I thought, "*What a butthead! He thinks MY nose is big!*" Today, Don says this was all part of a master plan to get me to notice him and to date him eventually three years later. I still don't buy it.

Okay, so it wasn't exactly love at first sight. The love came later. In high school, we became friends; in our junior year we started dating. Both of us were athletic and competitive. I was on the soccer team and Don was on the football, track and wrestling teams. Together we threw the football around and went wakeboarding on the lake behind my parents' house. But it was soccer that kept me from the homecoming dance in our junior year (broken ankle in three places). It was football that kept Don from the homecoming dance in our senior year (broken ankle). You could say it was fate!

Don and I shared many of the same friends; he became part of my family, coming over for dinner, talking with my parents, playing with my little sister Chia—even letting her do pull-ups on his arms. When it was time for college, he chose Colby in Maine while I chose Boston University. Although we loved each other, we decided to take a break and focus on the college experience. When we finished college, I moved back to Tampa to pursue a law degree and MBA from Stetson University. Don also moved back to Tampa, to earn his MBA at University of Tampa. That's when we started dating again.

After being together for several years, Don proposed in 2005. The time and place he chose for this were unusual, yet perfect. Don and I were scuba dive buddies, so at the end of one particular dive, we gathered at the bottom of the mooring line attached to the boat and prepared to surface. I looked down to check my depth and my air gauges; when I looked up, Don was holding an open box in front of me. Something in the box caught the sunlight and sparkled. I looked closer and realized it was a ring. I screamed… inside my regulator, of course. The ring was beautiful! Of course, being the big talker that I am, I found it difficult to experience one of my most life-altering moments under water, a place where I was unable to talk! (In a later conversation with Don, he joked that his reason for proposing under water was to ensure I didn't run away.)

After the proposal, my family members all swam up to Don and me, giving us underwater hugs. Six people in diving vests, masks, regulators and air tanks tried desperately to coordinate a group hug. When Don and I emerged from the Caribbean as an engaged couple, we continued our blissful vacation. I can still remember how excited I was. The man I was going to marry was someone I had grown up with. He knew me inside and out. He was caring, selfless, fearless and strong. He was my best friend; we shared the same life goals. I couldn't wait to spend the rest of my life with him. Don and I were married on October 28, 2006, celebrating at a reception at a St. Petersburg Beach hotel. We shared these moments with family and friends, including those who came from out of town and from out of the country. It was the happiest day of my life.

Soon after, we bought a little house in the neighborhood where I had grown up—a safe place, with huge oaks shading the sidewalks, magnolia trees, joggers, dogwalkers in the evening, children playing in their driveways. It was the perfect place to raise a family, yet close enough to Tampa's night life if we wanted to go out with friends. The "perfect place" was a great starter house, needing a bit of work but with enough room for a family, a pool, and a back yard for our dog, Tai. Tai was a lovable black boxer with droopy eyes, a goofy personality and a stump tail that never stopped wagging. Because our starter home was a bit dark and outdated, we wanted to bring light into it. My dad, who loves architecture, helped us remodel the house, and created a beautiful, bright, airy and welcoming place to live.

I loved our new home. I could picture our lives unfolding here, with scenes of dinner parties and barbecues with friends, our children learning to swim in the pool, Tai running in the yard, and out-of-town guests staying in our spare bedroom. Don and I were so happy there. Little did we know that our beautiful new home would deliver misery that would change the course of our lives.

Two years later, we found out that I was pregnant! We were so excited; we regarded this pregnancy as the third big step in our new lives together that started with our marriage and our new house. A while into my pregnancy, we received painful news: Tai, our dog, had cancer. This was a big blow to us because Tai was like our first child. Tai was the one who woke us up in the mornings by placing his paw on one of our hands and licking it. He greeted us at the door every day when we came home from work, trotted at our heels when we walked around the house, and cuddled with us.

Seeking a cure for Tai, we paid for his chemotherapy, which according to the veterinarian was not painful for dogs. Unfortunately, the chemo did not save him. Our goofy, kind-spirited, four-legged shadow died. Don and I were hit hard. The fact that we had a baby to look forward to eased the pain of Tai's loss.

By this time, Don was working long hours at his consulting job. As a trial attorney, I had just been made partner at a medium-sized law firm in Tampa. We were faced with the challenge of strategizing on how to raise children and maintain our careers at the same time. Would we hire a nanny to help out? Would we find good enough day care? What if the waiting list for a good day care facility was too long? Would we ask for help from our parents? We both worked 60–70 hours per week, so which of us would work fewer hours to care for our child? It was pretty overwhelming to us then.

When I think back to that time, those were such nice problems to have. It's funny how life alters one's perspective so quickly. Aside from strategizing about work and childcare, it was an exciting time for us. After we learned our baby was a boy, we had a lot of fun planning for him. Don, a former college football player, talked about how he would teach his son to play football. I planned the nursery with my mom and sister; my artistically talented mom and aunt were planning to paint cartoon images on the walls to match the bedding. Don and I couldn't wait to meet our son.

A little over five months into my pregnancy, I went into premature labor. This was obviously the last thing I expected to happen. My mind alternated between shock over the incident and worry that my premature baby would be all right. I desperately hoped that something could be done to stop the labor. When I arrived at the hospital, I learned that I was too far along in my labor for the process to be stopped. By the time I was hooked up to all the necessary machines, I learned that my baby did not have a heartbeat. He had died. A vice grip took hold of my stomach, twisting me up inside. My physical pain, sadness, and shock competed for my attention like wolves attacking helpless prey.

Every time the labor pains subsided, sadness swept over me, only to be beaten down again by more labor pains, only to be followed by shock; the cycle continued. I felt weak, sweating a lot. The whole event felt like an out-of-body experience. I could almost visualize my body lying on the table, being touched and prodded by medical staff. Everyone around me was talking but I don't remember what they said; I doubt I even recognized the words coming out of their mouths at the time. I felt so detached from the situation, as though it all happened in a hazy dream to someone else. Of course, my labor pains attacked me, shoving me into the fire that was reality. Every time the pains came, I had no doubt they were very real and happening to me. When the pains subsided, I faded back into the shock-induced haze, becoming detached, only to be delivered back to hell again by the returning pain. The cycle was relentless.

I remember the beeping, lots of beeping. Other than all of the above, the experience was a blur. After all the pain, the sweating, and the pushing, I gave birth to a premature, deformed, stillborn baby. Don was there with me, along with my family. All of them were loving and supportive, but I still felt completely alone, in utter shock.

After the birth, the doctor came to speak with us, explaining that the baby was dwarfed, among many other deformities, and would not have survived long after birth, even if he had lived for the entire pregnancy. This had happened inside of me; I had no idea why, and I was petrified. Was my body responsible or was it something else? Was it something I did? Over and over again I replayed my entire pregnancy in my mind, looking for something I could have done to cause this. I had never touched alcohol. I did not drink one sip of caffeine. I had taken no medicines, either prescription or over the counter. I had stayed away from all the foods that the doctor had told me not to eat. I stopped running, replacing that with speed walking; I kept my heart rate within the prescribed parameters. I ate very healthy unprocessed foods; I slept enough. How did this happen? Was it genetic? Both Don and I are familiar with several generations of our family lineage; neither of us had relatives or ancestors with dwarfism or any other deformities. This all didn't make sense to me.

A part of me had died and been torn out, both literally and figuratively. I felt empty. I didn't know what would fill that empty space again. I kept telling myself that I would have more children, but that would not change what had happened. We requested genetic testing; the results came back negative for genetic deformities. The cause was environmental then…but what was it? In the days following, I took time off from work, spending the time reading a lot and crying a lot. I was upset with myself for not being able to keep it together. I had always been tough, according to those who knew me best. I was emotionally strong, very independent, and rarely cried. I had always felt completely in control of my life; suddenly I felt helpless.

After returning to work, I had periods of feeling fine; then overwhelming sadness and crying fits would strangle me, holding me hostage at the most inconvenient times, which continued to frustrate me. I gave myself angry, drill sergeant-style pep talks to break myself out of it; nothing worked. I tried to drown out the sadness by focusing on my work. Just when I began to cope with the loss of the baby, I began to unravel the mystery of the strange symptoms I was experiencing.

In retrospect, I experienced ALS warning signs about one year before my pregnancy. I noticed problems with balancing and going down stairs. I would descend stairs slowly, holding the handrail, looking at my feet to make sure they were landing in the right place. The first time I realized that this was what I was doing—and that it wasn't normal—was when I saw my dad descend a flight of stairs. I told him, "Wow! You go down those stairs so fast, without even looking!" He looked at me oddly as if what he was doing was normal.

I also had an issue with running and skating. I used to run regularly. I would end my long distance run with a sprint, and I always tripped at the end. I thought it was because I pushed myself to my maximum ability and was merely too tired to maintain coordination. Additionally, I noticed a problem when skating. At one point, I went skating with a group of friends but found that it was difficult to balance and to move my legs in proper rhythm.

During pregnancy, I also had an issue with dancing. I was at my godson's christening, which involved Greek dancing. When I began to dance one particular Greek dance that I knew well, my legs seemed to have weights on them; I couldn't keep up with the speed of everyone else's dancing. When I asked my doctor whether my legs felt heavy was normal in pregnancy, he said he had never heard of it. He said that every woman experienced pregnancy differently so it could be possible that pregnancy had something to do with it.

One morning, as I was putting on my pants to go to work, I lost my balance. I caught myself by putting my foot out in front of me. I remembered another incident that occurred a few weeks later. I had lost my balance, falling over completely in my closet. I leaned over to pull my pants up, falling headfirst into a pile of dirty clothes, with my pants around my ankles and my behind sticking straight up in the air. At that moment Don came in, and said: "Well, Babe, I knew it annoyed you when I left the toilet seat up, but I don't think I deserve to be mooned for it!" I answered him with sarcasm, of course. "I'm modeling my new underwear. Be supportive!"

I laughed at my clumsiness, never suspecting that I had a serious disease. I told my dad about my recent loss of balance thinking the story was funny, but he was concerned and examined me. The examination revealed my reflexes were very hyperactive. My dad said that I needed to see a neurologist. The neurologist told me it was probably nothing serious, but he recommended that I have tests done. We had to delay my testing with the exception of an MRI of the brain until my second trimester, due to potentially harmful effects to the fetus. The MRI on my brain was done, and everything looked normal, which was encouraging. All other tests were postponed due to the pregnancy. Three weeks after I lost the baby, I visited the neurologist and he proceeded with the testing.

After I watched a movie with a character that had ALS, I was prompted to research the symptoms of ALS. When I found my symptoms were the same as those found in ALS, I freaked out. Two days later, I had the lumbar puncture, but the results were normal. The doctor called to ease my concerns, saying he really didn't think I had ALS, which put my mind at ease for the moment. Then, I received a nerve conduction test, and these results were also normal. This lulled me into a false sense of security.

An EMG study was to be performed, I knew the EMG would involve a lot of needles, which I can't stand. Don was out of town, so I decided to bring my dad. It made me more comfortable to have him there, and I knew he would talk to me and would distract me from the pain.

After the test was done, I remember sitting in the room with my dad, waiting for the neurologist. When he came into the room, he shook our hands and sat down. "The results of the tests show that you likely have ALS," he said with a poker face. Wait, I thought you said I didn't have ALS. The doctor said he was mistaken. I was in shock. I'm too young for this, I thought. The age range is 40 to 50. My heart pounded furiously, drowning out the sound of his voice. I knew all too well what the endpoint of ALS was. My close friend's father had ALS and he had died within five years of diagnosis. I didn't want my family to go through this. The doctor said, "There is a spectrum. At one end there is Primary Lateral Sclerosis (PLS) and at the other end, there is Amyotrophic Lateral Sclerosis (ALS). I believe you are close to the ALS side of the spectrum." The nausea creeping up inside me was relentless. The feeling was surreal. I looked around the room at the walls, the door, the doctor's chair, my chair, the doctor, my dad, my tightly clasped hands in my lap. I was here, on Earth. Everything around me was real. This nightmare was not a dream.

"What is the treatment? What does this mean for her?" my dad asked. My dad kept remarkably calm during the whole ordeal. The doctor replied, "There are treatments that can extend her life for a few months such as…" I didn't hear anything he recommended after saying the treatment could extend my life for only a few months. What that meant to me was there was no treatment. After my mind came back, I heard the doctor say, "…But you know, science progresses every day. There are always new studies and clinical trials being done at some of the most reputable institutions in the world…" I tuned out again. There were always new studies being done. I felt as though this was something that doctors with good bedside manners would say to avoid completely crushing people's spirits and evoking extreme emotional reactions from them and their families. I caught the tail end of his monologue, "…and I encourage you to seek multiple opinions."

He encouraged me to get multiple opinions. To me, that statement was my life raft in Class 5 white water. I clung to that life raft with white-knuckled terror while desperately trying to find a safe, dry piece of land to rescue me from this nightmare. As my dad drove me home from my appointment, I immediately began talking myself out of the fact that I had ALS. I raked my memory to find every single story I had heard and every article I had read about people who were told they had terminal illnesses, found out they were misdiagnosed, and lived happily ever after. I relayed those stories out loud to my dad as if these stories somehow made it less likely that I had ALS.

I'll tell you one thing, this is one freakishly wide and

long river. Even today I'm still floating, twirling, and being knocked around in it; I never seem to find my dry land. Is it exhausting? Yes. Am I afraid? No. I know that, one day, I'll find my land and I'll be proud of the challenge I conquered. To me, this is what hope looks like.

Chapter Two

Vince

I am Deanna's father and a retired orthopedic surgeon. I am my family's doctor. So, before seeing any neurologists, Deanna approached me and discussed her neurological symptoms. She explained that she tripped while running, felt awkward on stairs, had trouble dancing and lost her balance. I tested her reflexes, and they were definitely hyperactive. I remember using my reflex hammer and striking her patella tendon. Her leg shot up much faster than a normal reflex response. I reviewed her symptoms in my head. Immediately, ALS came to my mind. I thought back to my medical school days. I remembered my textbooks, which explained ALS in depth. What's strange is that those chapters on ALS were the only chapters in my medical books that I did not want to read. I remember reading the first few paragraphs and being overwhelmed by how horrendous the disease was. I couldn't even bear reading the text about it, and now my own daughter had it. Perhaps, my reaction in medical school was some sort of a premonition.

Whenever I thought about Deanna having ALS, I came up with every reason imaginable to discredit my initial suspicions. I'm an orthopedic surgeon, not a neurologist. I could be mistaken. What do I know? There are plenty of other neurological conditions with the same symptoms;

some that I probably don't even know exist. It could be something minor. Had Deanna not been my daughter, my emotions would never have prevented me from seeing objectively. Deanna's symptoms are the classic symptoms of a patient with ALS that first presents in the extremities. Even though I allowed myself to rationalize, I instructed Deanna to schedule an appointment with a neurologist and to have tests done.

At first the tests were negative, the first diagnosis that Deanna received was equivocal, PLS or ALS. Based on the symptoms that I observed in Deanna, I felt the condition was progressing too quickly to be PLS. Of course, I hoped I was wrong. Now, I know how many other conditions can cause similar symptoms to appear, Lyme's disease, for example. But at the time, both PLS and ALS scared me so much, that I just hoped Deanna had something else that was treatable. After Deanna received her ambiguous diagnosis, I began to search for a neurologist who could offer a second opinion. I asked a few neurologist colleagues of mine and they recommended a female physician who was Deanna's age.

To protect the doctor's identity, I'll call her Dr. Carter, which is not her name. Dr. Carter apparently had been the top performing physician in her residency program and had been noted for doing great work ever since graduating. I really thought she would be good for Deanna. Being a contemporary of Deanna's, Dr. Carter would likely understand and relate to Deanna better, which was important when dealing with such a tough diagnosis. I thought we were very lucky to have such a top performer available to Deanna in our region.

I visited Dr. Carter with Deanna. She was an intelligent, compassionate, and cheerful lady who spent a good deal of time with us. Deanna asked her "Do I have ALS?" Dr. Carter answered "Well, I'm not prepared to diagnose you until I see how you progress." It was inconclusive. Actually, this wasn't true, as Deanna later discovered from her medical records. Dr. Carter diagnosed ALS from the beginning. Why she didn't tell her, I don't know.

We were still waiting for a conclusive diagnosis. On the one hand, it was comforting to hear that Dr. Carter was not completely sure whether Deanna had ALS. On the other hand, not having an answer was incredibly nerve wracking. Deanna, I, and the rest of the family were waiting on the edges of our seats. A few weeks later, Deanna visited Dr. Carter again with Don, her husband. Still, Dr. Carter gave Deanna no unequivocal diagnosis.

All of us continued to hope for the best, but I could not stop thinking about Deanna's diagnosis, PLS or ALS. PLS is a much less aggressive form of ALS with the exact same outcome and impact on the body. PLS just progresses much more slowly. If Deanna does have ALS, even if she has the less aggressive PLS, why does she have it? There are two forms of ALS, sporadic and genetic. She definitely does not have the genetic version of ALS. Nobody in my family or Hedy's family has ever had any nerve condition, no siblings, parents, grandparents, great grandparents... so Deanna's ALS is, then, sporadic...but why? I couldn't quiet my mind. Why my daughter? I began to focus on this question intently; nothing could draw my attention away from finding an answer. I am sure that every ALS patient wants an answer to this question.

I researched and pulled every piece of medical literature I could find on sporadic ALS and its cause. I read through every one of these papers with an intensity and speed I had never felt before. I was in the zone. For every second it took me to read, that was one more second that my daughter's body was dying. I insist on printing things out rather than reading electronic copies. You can probably imagine what my office looked like a few days into my reading frenzy. There is an abundance of literature linking toxins to ALS. Forgive me for not referencing them all here.

Also, there are much higher instances of sporadic ALS in certain populations than in others. Multiple studies found that men with military service, in the last century, have a sixty percent greater risk of developing sporadic ALS than men who did not serve. Italian professional soccer players get sporadic ALS at a rate six times higher than that of the general population. Three teachers contracted sporadic ALS within a few decades, and their only commonality was that they taught in the exact same classroom. Now, three teachers may not seem like a large cluster, but it is an inexplicable cluster of cases, when three women contract the same, very rare disease in the same place and in a relatively short period of time. Statistically, these clusters of teachers, soccer players and soldiers are not likely to be coincidences.[2] If there are clusters, then there must be some external, environmental factor that triggers or causes sporadic ALS in these clusters. It is a clue that begs for a solution. Could it be viral? Could it be toxins? I needed more research.

I researched the available literature all day long and at night. Sometimes, I was able to get unpublished research from scientists or colleagues who were happy to help. I usually stopped at midnight and was up again at 4:00 a.m., woken by new ideas about the link between sporadic ALS and external factors. The studies all pointed to a common trigger. Every study agreed that these clusters were likely triggered by exposure to toxins. However, the research was frustratingly unclear on how toxins can cause ALS in some people and not in others. In fact, a text book on toxicology, *Casarett and Doull's*,[3] lists many toxins that can cause nerve degeneration. I was determined to find out if there was a link between toxins and Deanna's ALS. I asked Deanna many questions to try to find out whether she had been exposed to toxins. I asked her about what she had eaten, about what chemicals and personal care products she used at home, etc. We found nothing of concern.

---

2   Hyser, C.L., Kissel, J. T., Mendell, J. R. (1987). Three Cases of Amyotrophic Lateral Sclerosis in a Common Occupational Environment. *Journal of Neurology*, 234(6):443–4. http://www.ncbi.nlm.nih.gov/pubmed/3655851.

3   *Casarett & Doull's Toxicology: The Basic Science of Poisons*, 8th Ed. (2013).

Then, I came across a report on Chinese drywall. I investigated further and I found that there were countless lawsuits from people who had lived in houses with Chinese drywall. I found many reports. People who were young and otherwise healthy were reporting all sorts of health problems. Some of the people reported severe irreversible health issues; others reported problems such as upper respiratory symptoms.[4] ALS is a rare disease. So, I didn't see a link between Chinese drywall and ALS, at first.

I learned that, due to a few rough hurricane seasons, there was a domestic drywall shortage in the United States from 2005–2008, due to heavy reconstruction in damaged areas. The U.S. imported drywall from China. This Chinese drywall contained toxins, which were thought to be the cause of these reported health issues.[5] American drywall is not poisonous, as far as we know. Houses in Florida, Alabama, Mississippi, Louisiana, Virginia, and Southeast Texas that had been remodeled or built between 2005 and 2008 were at risk for having Chinese drywall because those were the states to which the imported drywall was shipped. The reports I read on Chinese drywall gave details about

---

4   Hooper, D. G., Shane, J., Straus, D.C., Kilburn, K.H., Bolton, V., Sutton, J.S., and Guilford, F.T. (2010). Isolation of Sulfur Reducing and Oxidizing Bacteria Found in Contaminated Drywall, *Int J Mol Sci—11(2), 647–655.* http://dx.doi.org/10.3390%2Fijms11020647.

5   CSPC-EPA Press Statement on Initial Chinese Drywall Studies. http://www.cpsc.gov//PageFiles/114254/oct2009statement.pdf; EPA Drywall Sampling Analysis, http://www.epa.gov/oswer/docs/chinesedrywall.pdf.

health problems found in people who were living in houses with Chinese drywall.

Having had toxins and ALS on my mind already, I immediately thought of Deanna's house in Florida, which had been remodeled in 2005. I began to research looking for more possible signs that there might be Chinese drywall in the house. According to studies on houses with Chinese drywall, copper tarnishes very quickly, a persistent smell of chemicals pervades the house, and people and animals experience respiratory and other health complications. I read the list out loud "copper tarnishing, chemical smell, health problems…" This was a connection. Deanna had mentioned these same symptoms in the home that she and Don had remodeled. I recalled Deanna's dog, Tai, getting cancer and dying. I thought of her unborn baby's deformities, and I found a connection between the high levels of strontium found in Chinese drywall and apparent dwarfism. I considered my son-in-law Don's health problems. When Don lived in the house, he constantly had upper respiratory problems. It seemed that there was never a time that he wasn't sick. He had never been sick this frequently during any other time in his life, according to him. Upper respiratory issues were some of the health issues caused by Chinese drywall. I picked up the phone to call Don.

Don understood the implications, and went into the attic. Sure enough, there was a stamp on the back side of the drywall that said "Made in China." Don took the covers off of several of the outlets in the house to check the wiring and it was corroded. He made another connection;

he and Deanna had noticed a while back that brand new mirrors in the house were tarnishing for no reason, which we later learned was another sign of toxic Chinese drywall. I recommended that Deanna and Don move out of their home, at least until we knew more about the situation. They moved in with Hedy and me. I really felt bad for them. I knew that the last thing a young newlywed couple wants to do is move in with their parents, but we had no other option at the time.

Don ripped off a piece of the drywall and sent it away to have it tested for toxins. The results confirmed my suspicions. The drywall in their house had disturbingly high levels of toxic metals.[6] The toxins present in elevated levels in Chinese drywall, such as strontium and sulfur compounds are harmful to humans when ingested and/or inhaled.[7] You may wonder how the toxic material in the drywall can end up poisoning people who live in a Chinese drywall house. When dry wall is sanded, it leaves a fine dust, much finer than normal dust. This dust floats

---

6   March 0f 2010 EMSL Analytical, Inc. completed testing of the drywall from Deanna and Don's home and reported more than eight times the concentration of lead and mercury in the Chinese drywall than in a control sample of U.S. drywall.

7   Hooper, D. G., Shane, J., Straus, D.C., Kilburn, K.H., Bolton, V., Sutton, J.S., and Guilford, F.T. (2010). Isolation of Sulfur Reducing and Oxidizing Bacteria Found in Contaminated Drywall, *Int J Mol Sci,* 11.2, 647–655. http://dx.doi.org/10.3390%2Fijms11020647; CSPC-EPA Press Statement on Initial Chinese Drywall Studies. http://www.cpsc. gov/PageFiles/114254/oct2009statement.pdf; EPA Drywall Sampling Analysis, http://www.epa.gov/oswer/docs/chinesedrywall.pdf.

around and constantly settles on surfaces, including in drinking glasses, on plates, in water, on the skin, etc. The drywall dust also becomes aerosolized in places where humidity is high, Florida is one of them. In humid conditions, when drywall dust is aerosolized, the particles are light enough to be carried by the air and never settle on surfaces. Instead, whoever lives in the house breathes the aerosol. In addition to these two factors, the drywall gives off gas, which is also inhaled. The drywall can emit a noxious sulfur-containing gas. For the toxins to be removed from a house, the Chinese drywall must be removed and any furniture or objects that collected drywall dust must be thrown away.[8] My daughter, her husband, their unborn baby and their dog had been inhaling and ingesting poison for years.

However, there was still one connection missing. The drywall may be the cause, I thought. But why does Deanna have ALS and not Don? I found an answer. Apparently, some people's bodies are better at eliminating toxins than others. Perhaps, athletes with low levels of body fat are more predisposed than others. Athletes, especially runners, soccer players and ballerinas, have little body fat. Body fat can trap toxins where the toxins remain without harm. If nerve or muscle cells are exposed to toxic substances degeneration of the cells can occur. That could explain athletes, soldiers, ballerinas and soccer players having clusters of ALS, if

---

8   CSPC-EPA Press Statement on Initial Chinese Drywall Studies. http://www.cpsc.gov//PageFiles/114254/oct2009statement.pdf.

exposed to toxins that trigger ALS. Those having difficulty trapping toxins in fat or eliminating toxins from their bodies are more likely to suffer permanent damage as a result of toxin exposure. ALS is rare and drawing conclusions is difficult. So, there might be other issues, too, but at least this was a starting place. I had found a plausible cause of Deanna's disease, but was this the cause of Deanna's ALS?

Returning to Deanna's unborn child, what could have caused the apparent dwarfism and other deformities? Strontium is one of the toxins known to be present at elevated levels in Chinese drywall.[9] When absorbed by the body, strontium fixes itself to the bone growth plates, replacing calcium in the bones.[10] At high enough concentrations, this causes bone growth to cease. Deanna's fetus had bones that were much shorter than they were supposed to be, making the doctor conclude that the baby suffered from Dwarfism, even though there was no evidence of genetic dwarfism in the fetus or in the family of

---

9   CSPC, Executive Summary of October 29, 2009 Release of Initial Chinese Drywall Studies (TABA). http://www.cpsc.gov/PageFiles/114760/TabA.pdf.

10   Hooper, D. G., Shane, J., Straus, D.C., Kilburn, K.H., Bolton, V., Sutton, J.S., and Guilford, F.T. (2010). Isolation of Sulfur Reducing and Oxidizing Bacteria Found in Contaminated Drywall, *Int J Mol Sci, 11.2, 647–655.* http://dx.doi.org/10.3390%2Fijms11020647; Matsumoto. A. (1976). Effect of Strontium on The Epiphyseal Cartilage Plate Of Rat Tibiae-Histological And Radiographic Studies. *Japanese Journal of Pharmacology, 26.6, 675–81.* http://www.ncbi.nlm.nih.gov/pubmed/1021603; EPA Drywall Sampling Analysis. http://www.epa.gov/oswer/docs/chinesedrywall.pdf.

either Deanna or Don. I believe that strontium in the Chinese drywall caused the apparent dwarfism and death of her unborn baby.

I wanted Deanna to be tested for toxins. I began to read toxicology and medical literature about toxin testing to see what types of tests could be done on Deanna. I found out that toxins can be present in the blood or can be fixed in other tissues. Fixed toxins can be anywhere, in nerve tissue, fat, bones, or other places, depending on the toxins. Only fat and red blood cell samples can be tested with testing methods available for living patients. I wanted to test Deanna's blood and fat tissue for toxins. I knew that if the toxins were fixed elsewhere in Deanna's body, then the tests would come back negative. Nevertheless, I was determined to know what we could know about Deanna's exposure to toxins from the Chinese drywall.

With my new knowledge of the link between ALS and toxins and the information about the particular toxins in the Chinese drywall in Deanna's home, I was eager to go to Deanna's neurologist. I wanted to approach Dr. Carter with what I had found. I was eager to speak with her doctor about the link between the toxins in Deanna's house and her ALS.

I brought up the idea of toxins being connected to ALS with Dr. Carter. "Doctor," I asked, "what are your thoughts about toxins as the cause of ALS? I found in my research that it's widely accepted in the neurology community that toxins can be a trigger for ALS." Let me interject here that neurologists will readily admit that toxins can be a "trigger" for ALS but are reluctant to say that they may be a "cause." This is a very superficial distinction which makes no sense to me. Neurology textbooks classify toxins as a possible cause for neural degeneration. I explained, "If Deanna has ALS, she definitely doesn't have familial ALS, and she was living in a house with Chinese drywall for two and a half years. There were high levels of aluminum, strontium, sulfur, mercury, lead and cadmium in the drywall, when it was tested. She had been breathing those toxins for two and a half years. I think that the toxins may be connected to her disease, whether it's ALS or PLS. They may also be the reason for the dwarfed fetus and..."

She interrupted and impatiently said "You think toxins could be the cause..."

I continued to explain myself. "Yes, strontium replaces calcium in bone and stops the bones from growing. There were high levels of strontium in Deanna's drywall. Her fetus was dwarfed with no genetic history of dwarfism in either our family or Don's family and they both tested negative genetically for a gene mutation for dwarfism. That leads me to believe the cause was environmental."

"You don't know that," she curtly interrupted. I was taken aback. I thought to myself, "Is this the same doctor I met the first time Deanna came here?" My mention of toxins and continued explanation of my reasons for my belief seemed to trigger a personality transformation in this good doctor. I was shocked. I tried one more time to reason with Dr. Carter. "Neurology and toxicology textbooks clearly state that toxins are a trigger for nerve degeneration. That's an undisputed fact. It seems that if this is the case, they certainly can be a cause. They're certainly not safe. She's moved out of her house because the exposure to…"

She didn't wait for me to finish. "There is no reason for her to move out of her house. There is absolutely no proof that toxins can cause ALS."

"But Doctor," I interjected. "It is a known fact that they trigger nerve degeneration. I'm not sure how anyone can conclude that there is no proof that they can be a cause."

An obviously annoyed Dr. Carter repeated herself. "There is no proof that they are a cause for ALS."

"OK," I answered, because I was making no headway, "but you do acknowledge that they are a trigger for nerve degeneration?"

"Yes," She answered. "But that does not prove that they are a cause."

Ahhh, finally some progress, and I continued, "Will you at least agree that toxins are dangerous, due to the fact that they trigger nerve degeneration? That seems like a logical assumption…which is why she moved out of her house."

"There is no need for her to move out of her house." She answered abruptly.

I was floored. This statement was completely illogical to me. Toxins are known to cause nerves to die, but she would not admit that they could be a cause for diseases that cause the nerves to die. That's like saying that smoking cigarettes harms the lungs, but then saying that there is no proof that smoking causes lung disease. "Well," I continued, "I would like to find more out. Is there a way that you can test her blood and fat cells for toxins?" I asked a few more questions, which Dr. Carter answered only with distain. "Listen, I'm not a toxicologist and I don't really see the point of testing for toxins."

"I realize you're not a toxicologist, but I feel that finding a cause for the disease is important. If the drywall is the cause, we may be able to find a way to remove the toxins from her body and interfere with the disease process."

This time, Dr. Carter not only cut me off, again, and stated "I'm not going to test for toxins, and there is no way to interfere with the disease process. Motor Neuron Diseases don't have a cure. I know it's hard to hear, but that's the truth."

I thought when did this type of attitude from a professional become OK? Allow me to interject. As I previously stated, I found in my research that the neurology community widely accepts that toxins can be a trigger for ALS. Neurologists will readily admit that toxins are a trigger, but are reluctant to call toxins a cause. A trigger and a cause are virtually one in the same. It frustrates me that neurologists flatly deny any cause and effect relationship, when toxicology textbooks make this claim, clearly. Don't neurologists and toxicologists talk?

I said, "If you think of anything that may be of use or have any ideas...or change your mind about testing for toxins for that matter, please contact me."

The next morning, I was drinking my coffee and checking my email. I opened my inbox and I was absolutely delighted to see an email from Dr. Carter. Perfect! She's changed her mind! She wants to help us! I looked up at the ceiling and said "Thank you!" I don't know who I was thanking...perhaps God or my parents, grandparents, or any other deceased relatives whom I hoped were floating around watching over my family. I opened the email. By this time, I had become so emotionally involved in Deanna's disease already and there was no turning back. Anyway, I no longer have the email from Dr. Carter, so I can't tell you word for word what it said, but it read like this:

Vince,

I appreciate your concern about your daughter's health, but I am her physician and I would appreciate if you would leave the job to me. I understand that you're her dad and want to help, but she is an adult and you are not doing any good butting in. You are emotional and you are a bleeding heart, which is not helping her at all. You are doing severe and irreparable psychological damage to your daughter and to yourself by looking for the cause of this disease and giving her false hope that there may be a solution to her problems. Motor Neuron Disease is not curable and it is fatal. There is no other case to argue. These are the facts. I would appreciate it very much if you would discontinue your involvement in your daughter's medical affairs, for her sake. Again, you are harming her and, if you do not stop, she will not recover from this.

My heart fell to the floor. I read the email over and over again in disbelief. I can't believe this crap. I'm being reprimanded because I love my daughter and I'm trying to learn about her disease so I can help her. I had enough sense to treat her as a peer and regard her with respect, yet she spoke to me and wrote to me as though I was her underling—know-nothing pest, who was just complicating her job. What kind of a doctor tries to discourage another doctor from looking for the cause or solution to a problem? Who cares if I'm emotionally affected? This is my daughter. Hope is not false just because no treatment or cure has been found. Hope motivates people to find answers and solutions, to ask questions, and to gain new insights into the disease and to fight.

It is so difficult for me to understand the mindset of a young bright neurologist who completely lacks curiosity regarding possible treatment methods for ALS. How could she accept such a disastrous status quo with no desire to think outside of the box? I believe that this neurologist is the classic example of a victim of group think and didactic medicine. Accepting the status quo and the grim prognosis contributes nothing to medicine or to patients. The medical community has been trying to find an ALS treatment for over 200 years, to no avail. It's no surprise that neurologists have lost hope, but I'm a father and losing hope for my child, even if she is an adult, isn't an option for me. My life has taught me to challenge the status quo and to do what needs to be done, even if it is unconventional. If I know one thing that got me through life, it is to persevere. To never quit. I was not about to quit on Deanna, when she needed me.

In Dr. Carter's comments and in her voice, I heard the voices of all of those in my past who told me I couldn't achieve my goals. Dr. Carter's email made me angry, but it motivated me even more. Deanna will beat this, and she and I both will be sure to contact Dr. Carter when she does.

The first neurologist we saw recommended Deanna get multiple opinions so we sought an appointment at a very well-known ALS clinic.

Deanna and I went to the institution, the supposed Mecca of Neurology, along with my wife and Don. We sat in the room waiting for the doctor to come in, much like we did when we saw the previous doctor.

"There's a chance that it's not ALS." Deanna said. "The previous two doctors couldn't make the diagnosis, so there must be something different about me". She continued to speak looking at my face for reassurance. I nodded my head.

"You're right," I confirmed. "It is possible that it's not ALS."

"I feel fine. Some of my symptoms even disappear every once in a while." She eagerly looked at me again.

"Is that right?" I asked. I reached over, took her hand in mine.

Hedy rubbed her back and reassured her with a smile "let's see what he says. We'll figure this out together." I didn't know what to say to her. She was so hopeful and so were Hedy and I. As a physician, I knew what future was in store for someone with Motor Neuron Disease of any type and it wasn't good. With every statement Deanna made reassuring herself, she looked at me for confirmation, with a wide eyed hopefulness and innocence that she had grown out of many years ago. That look was back and stabbed and tore at the pit of my stomach; it was merciless. This time, I couldn't offer her any hope or confirmation. I was blank. My baby girl needed me, and I had nothing. Those hopeful eyes reminded me of my worthlessness every time they looked at me.

So many memories came flooding back to me of Deanna when she actually was my baby girl. I drifted off into never land re-experiencing her childhood. I couldn't help it; that look was haunting me. Deanna was always small for her age, with a huge personality. She loved to dress up in costumes and imitate the adults around her while exaggerating their idiosyncrasies. She would sit in my favorite chair with my bathrobe on over her clothes. The robe would drag on the floor and her feet would barely reach the edge of the seat of the chair when she sat back in it. That's how tiny she was. She would sit with my robe and watch on and pretend to read the paper while she parroted comments I always made while reading the news usually about finance, crime, or politics. She mimicked me in the best male voice and New York accent that she could muster up with her tiny squeaky vocal chords.

Deanna always hated to be told she couldn't do something because she was too small, too young, too weak, or not ready. Her lips would purse, her freckly nose would crinkle, her rodent-sized marker stained hands would roll into tiny white knuckled fists, and she would not stop trying until she proved us all wrong. She almost never wanted help, but if she was really having trouble she would let her tough-girl façade down and show me her soft side. When she needed me, she would give me that look, the same one I saw in the waiting room at the doctor's office...those big green eyes, full of hope. "Daddy, I have a cut. Can you fix it?" "Daddy, I'm scared." "Can you help me?" "Daddy, I just can't do it. Can you show me how?" I was always the one with an answer. When I did, she looked at me, eyes sparkling with amazement, like I was a real live super hero.

"Dad" I heard her voice. She, Don, and Hedy stood up to greet the doctor who had walked in while I was busy walking down memory lane. The doctor was tall and thin with dark hair, rounded shoulders, and pale skin. "Hi" I greeted him. "Vince Tedone." He gave me a cold fish handshake and made no expression. We shook hands and we all sat down. Deanna watched his expressionless face eager for some clue about what her diagnosis would be. He asked Deanna questions in his monotone voice as if he were reading from a script; he never looked her in the eye. He looked at her charts and clicked on several boxes on his computer. After a while, he finally turned to look at Deanna.

"It appears that you have ALS." There was no emotion in his voice, no sorrow and no attempt to show empathy or respect that she was receiving devastating news, just a matter of fact statement. The stabbing feeling in the pit of my stomach, brought forth by Deanna's hopeful look, became stronger. My heart pounded. My mouth felt dry. I looked at Deanna. She shuttered in disbelief. Her eyes watered and her trembling hand rose to cover her mouth. She gained composure quickly. I looked at Hedy; she was breathing heavily, but maintained her poker face and put an arm around Deanna.

"OK," she said. "Well, what can I do? How can I beat this? I've been exercising the areas of my body that are weaker to keep them strong. What else is there?"

"Well," he answered. "There's not much you can do. Exercise isn't a good idea because if you tire out your muscles, they may waste away faster and not come back."

"But won't being sedentary and not moving at all also cause muscle wasting? I mean, that causes muscles to weaken in normal people; wouldn't it do the same for someone with ALS?"

He didn't acknowledge her question and interjected impatiently. "Do you use a cane to walk?" he asked.

"No" Deanna answered him.

"You will; and after that, you'll need a wheelchair and you'll eventually be bed ridden."

Her face turned white and her eyes widened. Deanna quickly erased the look and replaced it with a polite one, which amazed me. She maintained her composure much better than most people I know could have; just like her mother. She had such grace. "Oh…OK…" She said politely.

She smiled, nodded, and said "Th...thank you." Her voice quivered and she was fighting back tears.

"I see the disease has already affected your voice..."

"No..." She quietly interrupted him. "I...I'm just upset...I'm...this is...uh...hard news to receive. I speak just fine and..."

"It's affected your voice." He interrupted. "It is what it is. You'll eventually lose your ability to speak, so you should have your voice recorded so you can speak with a computer, which you'll eventually control with your eyes because your hands will become paralyzed."

"Oh," She said politely while forcing another smile and nodding. Unbelievable! I thought. She's so sweet, polite, and composed! He's just massacring her without any sign of remorse! Hedy shook her head and I interjected. I couldn't help myself.

"Excuse me, doctor. I understand the prognosis, but the disease has not affected her voice. I talk to her all the time. Her voice is fine."

"Whether it has or not is not even important." He answered with a frustrated tone. "It will, so she needs to prepare for it."

"No..." Deanna's brows furrowed, she leaned back in her seat, and her trembling hand rose to cover her mouth once again. I put my arm around her. "Not my voice." She sounded bewildered. "How will I...how will I work?"

The doctor shook his head. "Are you still working? You shouldn't be. You won't be able to after a while, so I suggest you just start enjoying your life now, while you're still mobile and can speak." I had had it with this man. Is he unable to process emotional cues? Does he have some sort of psychological syndrome that prevents him from feeling empathy? This guy isn't normal.

I asked the doctor, probably with a challenging tone "Have you ever had ALS patients who have performed exercises? Have you evaluated their effect on disease progression?"

"No." He answered.

"Then how do you know it's not helping her and that it can't help others?"

He ignored my question and addressed Deanna. "Do you have trouble eating? Do you choke easily?"

"No, not at all." Deanna answered. "That's a good sign, right?" My beautiful daughter still managed to muster up a smile for the doctor when she asked this question. Perhaps that smile was her last sliver of hope shining through.

"That means nothing. All it means is that the disease hasn't attacked that area of your body yet. You will eventually have to be on a liquid diet and then, in time, a feeding tube. It will only be a simple surgical procedure where they'll insert a tube into your intestines and feed you through there."

I could see the pain in my daughter's face. Her brows furrowed again, her forehead creased, and the corners of her mouth turned down. Her face was white.

"Is there anything we can do to prevent atrophy in other areas, like breathing exercises?" I asked.

"Deanna, are you having trouble breathing?" He continued, completely avoiding my question yet again.

"No, I breathe just fine. I can start doing breathing exercises...if it will help."

"You will eventually need a respirator. I wouldn't waste your time on exercises." I was furious! Is this guy emotionally inept?! I thought. As a physician, I understand the doctor's duty to stay emotionally detached, but not to this extent...he's unbelievable...inhuman!

"Doctor..." I was getting upset with him. "You've told her about all of the things she won't be able to do. How about focusing now on what she can she do? This disease has been studied for over 200 years; there must be something that we can do."

"Well, she can take Riluzole."

"So, there is a treatment" I tried to pull something of use out of him—anything.

"Yes, it will extend her life for two to three months. There are adverse side effects. Listen, he said, there is no cure for ALS. I realize you want to exercise and do things to slow the progression, but it just can't be done. Go home and enjoy your life while you can. The life expectancy for ALS is two to five years. Get your affairs in order because at the mid and latter stages of your disease, you'll be bedridden and won't be able to take care of your affairs. It's best to do it now." "There is no cure on the horizon." He stood up ready to leave.

"Look" I tried to find some ray of hope for Deanna. "I

have reason to believe that Deanna's ALS was caused by toxins in Chinese drywall. Can you test her for toxins?" "Toxins?" He seemed confused. "Yes, all of the medical literature on ALS confirms that toxins can cause motor nerve degeneration. She was exposed to high levels of toxins for two and a half years. The toxins are likely still in her body and if we can remove them..." He interrupted me mid-sentence. "I'm not a toxicologist. Even if we found toxins, I don't know what good that would do." "Well, is anyone at your institution trying to find out which toxins cause ALS?" He returned my look with a blank stare and gave an answer that was the most long winded version of "no" I had ever heard. "I have reports on the toxins in her house, if that would help." I tried desperately to force him to react. Again, he met me with a blank stare and a shake of the head.

"We can't test her for toxins." How is this possible? I thought. This institution is world renowned for the study of ALS and this man, supposedly an ALS God, is completely disinterested in finding out what causes the disease in the first place! Imagine if we did know what toxins cause ALS. Perhaps we could prevent ALS.

The doctor left the exam room. Deanna turned toward me with a defeated look said "The doctor said there is nothing that can be done." "What this guy is telling you is complete horse shit, excuse my language, but it's true. This is NOT the end. Do you hear me? This is the beginning." I saw a fragment of that hope come back to her face; I had brought it back. All I had to do was keep it there. We walked out of the doctor's office. We nicknamed that doctor "The Undertaker," and vowed never to see him again.

Unfortunately, when Deanna and I arrived home, we faced the difficult task of confronting our family with this news. Everyone in a family responds differently to bad news. After Deanna's diagnosis, nobody's life remained the same. We have been changed, forever.

Chapter Three

Don

I am Deanna's husband.

When I learned that Deanna had ALS, it was anti-climactic for me because all along I had a strong feeling her symptoms were caused by ALS. I had already started my grieving process. I'm not an emotional person, and I can't stay sad or worried for very long about things I can't control. When it comes to negative emotions, I tend to compartmentalize. I turn my feelings off, or cover them up, I should say, and I focus all of my energy on doing what I need to do to make the situation better.

I tried to think of ways that I could let Deanna know that I would be there for her and would never leave her side. Knowing her as well as I knew her, I predicted that she was going to try to convince me to leave. I tried to find ways to force the emotions out of her so she could cry on my shoulder. She's more the type to maintain composure than she is the type to let it all out emotionally. I wanted her to feel free to let it out; it wasn't healthy to hold it in.

I didn't believe that Deanna was going to die from this disease; I don't know why, but I didn't and this was before the Deanna Protocol® treatment came along. It was as if my subconscious knew something that my conscience didn't know yet. I knew ALS would disable Deanna and that she would need medication and care, so when I heard she had ALS, I immediately started strategizing and thinking logistically and financially about how I would care for her. I worried about how I would take care of Deanna and work at the same time. I already worked 70 hours a week as an information technology consultant for global companies. Working long hours is the norm among people in my career, so it's not like I could have found positions requiring me to work less. I thought about taking a different job, but then I realized that any job paying less wouldn't be a good idea because I would need the money; care and medication for an ALS patient can cost as much as raising two children, so I needed to keep my job, especially since Deanna might stop working.

Basically, when I found out that Deanna had ALS, my mind was full of contingency plans. As Deanna's physical condition started to decline, my mother-in-law and I became like her pit crew getting her ready for work every morning, helping her with clothes, shoes, legal files, etc. It was all hands on deck getting her ready for work and a big sigh of relief every morning when we managed to make sure she left on time. This was before the Deanna Protocol® was developed, of course, so she still had symptoms like spasticity, which would cause her to frequently drop things (shampoo in the shower, car keys, paper, you name it). You can imagine how this would make getting ready in the morning a nightmare for her. She would also freeze while walking, which also made the mornings challenging for her. She was more upset about needing us than we were about helping her. All of these things made getting ready in the morning an adventure to say the least. We were happy to help, and she was so upset that she had to ask. I just wanted Deanna to be happy and okay. That was my focus and whatever it took to do that, I would do.

One day, Deanna's dad called me about a possible link between drywall, toxins and Deanna's ALS. We had remodeled our home and put up some new walls. I went in the attic to see if I could tell from where the drywall came. There, on the back of the drywall, it read, MADE IN CHINA. Vince was convinced from his research that the toxins in Chinese drywall could have been a trigger for Deanna's ALS. He asked me to check the wiring for corrosion. I took off the electrical plates, and the copper wiring was corroded. The brand new mirrors were tarnishing for no reason, also. I sent some of the drywall off for testing, and the report came back showing high levels of heavy metals of all types, much higher than these levels should be in American drywall. We were making some progress, at last.

I probably seemed unemotional on the outside. However, I was sad and crying on the inside. This is how I deal with grief. I would like to think that my lack of emotional displays has provided Deanna some support. I would like to think I'm her rock...or one of her rocks at least. I am proud of Deanna's courage. I don't know what I would do without her.

Chapter Four

Hedy

I am Deanna's mom.

I was sitting in the doctor's office along with Deanna and my husband while the final examination took place. Until now, there had been no final diagnosis. We all made light hearted comments, including the doctor, and that gave me a false sense of security that there was really no serious problem. When the doctor was finished with the testing he stared at the computer for a while and then turned around and announced that he had very strong suspicions that Deanna has ALS. He continued telling her all of the terrible things that would happen to her as the disease would take hold of her body, section by section, and told her she had 2–5 years left of her life. "I suggest you make the best of it," he said. It was almost a routine speech, what was missing was "take some Aspirin and see me in a few days." He left to follow his office routine and we were left behind with earth shattering, life changing news.

This announcement took my breath away; I felt pressure assaulting my body from all sides, like I was being squeezed. My skin suddenly felt like a wet suit that was several sizes too small. I felt the need to remove it quickly before going crazy, which I know may seem odd. It was the strangest feeling I had ever had. Thoughts of Deanna and ALS were racing through my mind so quickly that I couldn't focus on a single one for enough time to feel sad. I was just in shock and numb. I remember hearing ringing in my ears too. My mouth went completely dry and I lost my speech. I tried to speak several times, but no words would come out. I wanted to comfort Deanna and say things that would ease the blow of this terrible diagnosis. I was completely mute...trapped in my own mind.

I wanted to get up from my chair to give Deanna a comforting, protective motherly hug, but I was rooted there like a statue and I could not. Eventually, I was able to reach out to her and put my arms around her. My reaction annoyed, confused, and surprised me. This was a time when she needed love and support the most and I just sat there and offered nothing. I feel like I failed her then. To this day, that moment haunts me and so does the guilt.

The day after the appointment, it really hit me that Deanna has ALS. The veil of shock somewhat lifted, the following nights were filled with tears and nonstop prayers. My mind was racing. I did not want to read about ALS. I had some knowledge, but I needed to stay away from more depressing news. I stayed away from the computer too. I had decided that it was my job to stay strong and to be a rock for Deanna, my husband, our daughters, our grandchildren, and the rest of the family. The last thing they needed was a weeping distressed mother to worry about. I put myself in charge of positive spins. Anything that was negative that I heard or that would happen, I would find a positive spin and stress that. I wanted positive energy to flow in and around all of us, especially Deanna.

I went into hyper-drive waiting on Vince and Deanna, so Vince would be completely free to research Deanna's condition and figure out what he could do for her. Deanna would feel less of a burden while she was going through this tough time. I did Deanna's laundry, cooked her breakfast, packed her lunch, and cooked her dinner. I cleaned up after her too. She must have thought I had gone crazy treating her like she was a child; she tried to stop me several times, but I insisted. If I wasn't doing this, what else could I do? I felt useless.

Since Deanna started the Deanna Protocol®, which came later in the game, I have been in charge of the medication. It's tough for her to unscrew pill bottles, sort pills, and write on the labels. She can do it, but it takes her much longer, so I took over. I sort about 300 pills a week and prepare her liquid medication too. I also make Deanna food to eat before and after taking her medication. For a long time, I hand made the pills by putting powder in tiny capsules. Before the Deanna Protocol®, when her physical condition was still declining, she lost some of her proprioception and feared losing her balance while walking. I went with her everywhere so she could hold on to me. I walked her around the house, to the car, to the bathroom, to bed, to the kitchen table, you name it, and I was there. When the cane and walker became an acceptable tool, she regained some of her independence.

Deanna can do most things herself but it takes a lot of time. Sometimes, there was not enough time in the day for that, so in order to speed up the process, I inserted myself wherever I could. I helped her get dressed, made her food, assisted with her hair, and her makeup, etc. My son-in-law, Don, and I got her purse and bags together, helped her with her shoes, and loaded her car every morning before work. I also was there to help her out of her car when she would come home and to help her make dinner, dress for bed, and complete her evening routine. Any way I could make things faster or easier for her, I would try. I admit that I hovered a lot; I guess that's how I dealt with my grief. Any time I was doing something for myself, running errands, or doing anything other than staying home and helping Deanna, I felt such terrible guilt. I felt like I was being a bad mother. I had this idea in my head that my every waking moment should be focused on Deanna and, if it wasn't, I was neglecting her. I have finally forced myself to let go a little bit and not hover so much, although it's very tough and I still fall back into hover mode from time to time. It took a long time rid myself of the guilty feeling I had any minute that I wasn't focusing on Deanna. It's still not completely gone; but its better and it's not torturous anymore, so that's good.

Most importantly what keeps me going is hope, faith, Deanna's sunny smile, positive attitude, and gratitude.

Chapter Five

Andrea

I am Deanna's sister, her older sister.

I know exactly where I was when I found out Deanna was diagnosed. It was mid-summer and my kids were in the middle of swim class in the back yard and the phone rang. I knew Deanna had been to the doctor to find out what was causing her strange symptoms and I was eager to find out if everything was okay. I assumed it was. I picked up the phone and heard my dad say "she has ALS." My legs became like bricks, my heart started pounding, and I was speechless. It felt like a truck hit me. My mind was racing. I was unable to process all that I already knew about the disease.

It was very ironic, actually. Not too long before that, Deanna had called me on the way to meet friends for dinner. "I know what I have," Deanna said matter of factly, "I have ALS." I told her she was crazy, but I didn't even know, exactly, what ALS was. So, I immediately went home and researched it. What I found was so horrifying, I kept convincing myself that she was just paranoid. Denial worked, until Dr. Vince Tedone, my dad, said "she has ALS."

I was in utter shock. Over the next several weeks, I found myself hiding in the bathroom crying so my children wouldn't see me. I would cry myself to sleep, I would wake in the middle of the night with racing thoughts, and I would cry again. My little sister, the one I had begged my parents for when I was a kid, the one who was my best buddy, my childhood side-kick, and my best friend was going to die. I felt HELPLESS. I can't imagine a worse feeling. I started seeing a therapist to help me get my arms around the situation. I needed to find a place where I could pull myself together for my children. The therapy helped me, and I recommend that to anyone in a similar situation.

I needed to turn the helplessness into hopefulness. So, I decided to put together a walk team for the ALS Association Tampa Chapter annual walk. I threw all of my energy into raising money for the walk. We had a staggering 50 walkers raising money. Our team "Winning the Fight" raised more money than any walk team had ever raised in Tampa and we were second that year for all walks in the State of Florida that year. The turn out and enthusiasm was not a testament to my hard work but a testament to how people feel about Deanna. We were all determined to do something for her.

Every once in a while, I still feel incredibly angry that Deanna has ALS. The anger overwhelms me. Sadness overcomes me, too. I still break down and cry, sometimes. Of course, I hide while I'm doing it so my kids don't see me. I worry a lot about my parents and the toll this is taking on them. I can't imagine their grief, pain, fear, sorrow and fatigue.

I want my children to know their grandparents, and I want my parents to see their grandchildren grow up. My parents have always been much younger than their age in terms of how they look, physical abilities/strength, and mental/physical health. I'm afraid that the stress of the disease has taken some of that away from them. I would love them to be there at my children's high-school and college graduations. By helping with Winning the Fight, Inc., I hope that I can do something to help Deanna and others struggling with ALS and to take some of the burden off of my parents.

Chapter Six

Chiara

I am Deanna's sister, the youngest of the three sisters.

I was 25 and living in Washington, D.C., when Deanna was finally diagnosed. My biggest worries were developing my career, studying for graduate school admissions tests, logging enough time at the gym every week, affording my overpriced shoe-box sized apartment in the city, and finding time for my social life. It's funny how it takes a tragedy to remind people of what's really important.

I remember finding out about Deanna's diagnosis. The memory is still so vivid to me. My phone was broken and I was at the Apple store waiting in a long line to get it fixed. The employees let me use their landline to call my dad, who scared me with his text saying "I need to talk to you. This is serious. You need to call me now." I called my dad and he told me, "Deanna has Motor Neuron Disease." I had no idea what was Motor Neuron Disease.

I asked if she could die from Motor Neuron Disease and my dad said "yes." I felt like I was missing a limb not having my cell phone available to Google "Motor Neuron Disease" and find out exactly what it was. We hung up the phone after talking and I felt in limbo. I didn't know whether I should be sad, scared, shocked, or if I should hold on to hope and forget the negative emotions.

I Googled Motor Neuron Disease later, but that didn't help. There were so many MNDs and she could have any of them, so I chose to believe that she had one of the least aggressive types. I didn't really start to become frightened until I came home to see my family for Thanksgiving. Deanna had declined dramatically since the last time I saw her. My denial set in then, followed by periods of realizing the truth, followed by denial, etc. My brain followed this cycle more times than I can count.

I flew to Tampa every five weeks to see my family. I would take Friday and sometimes half of Thursday off on the weeks that I flew home. This took a lot of planning and preparation. To make up for the time off, I put every effort into finishing projects very early so my absence wouldn't impact my work. Exceeding my deadlines by several days required me to maintain intense focus and work at an exhausting pace. Additionally, to make up for the hours I missed in the office, I usually spent several days arriving at the office at 5:00 am and working until 9:00 pm or sometimes later. Every time I came home, I would leave scared and shocked at how quickly Deanna had declined. I also would leave surprised at how much other members of my family had declined emotionally.

For almost two years, I continued this pattern of working long hours, barely sleeping, traveling home, and finding myself sad and in shock, and returning to D.C. drained of energy. I wanted to be home. Eventually, I had to admit to myself that, if I wanted to be near my family, I would have to switch careers and start an entirely new life. There were no jobs in my industry that would allow me to live in Tampa full time. I quit my job, moved home, and I worked as a nanny and a tutor while I decided on a new career path. I decided to pursue business, applied for an MBA program, and began taking classes. Leaving my career, my life in D.C., and my friends behind after nine years in the city was sad, but being away from my family felt much worse. The decision to start a new life was easy to make, but very tough to execute.

I am still building my new life. I'm still frightened for Deanna, although not as much because I believe Deanna will live, now that she's on the Deanna Protocol®. What frightens me the most *now* is what this disease is doing to my parents. They haven't had any opportunity to relax or enjoy their retirement. Retirement is supposed to be relaxing and carefree, but for them, it is tough, exhausting, frightening, and stressful.

Chapter Seven

Deanna's Disease Progression

I still remember my first day as a lawyer. I was 25 and fresh out of law school. With no work experience, I was ready to learn and ready to make my mark on the world. As a young baby-faced twenty-five year old female, I was entering into a field dominated by older men. I was confident in my ability to learn and succeed, but I was not without fear. Fear of uncertainty. I had no idea what was in store for me as an attorney, but I was more than eager to work as hard and long as necessary to be one of the best. When I looked at my desk on that first day in the office, I was already imagining myself forty years later, sitting at a larger desk in a grander office, wise with experience, having overcome adversity and basking in the glow of hard won success. I was imagining myself as a partner in a law firm, a founder of my own firm, or maybe as a judge, or an in-house counsel for a multi-national corporation. The options were plentiful and mine for the taking. This excited me!

I am now coping with ALS. At first, I didn't want to give up anything; juggling and trying to keep the balls in the air. Working sixty or seventy hours in a week, as an attorney, I was trying to keep up with my own expectations, and the expectations of my coworkers. There was no denying my physical limitations and the toll that ALS was taking on my body.

The inefficiency of my body made mundane tasks, previously completed without a second thought, a chore. I needed a lot of help just to get out the door on time in the morning. So, my analytical brain went to work, cataloging the inefficiencies and determining how I could become more efficient, despite the new limitations imposed by ALS. I was determined not to let a disease steal my dreams. However, things like trips between the bedroom and bathroom could take a lot of time, because I walked so slowly. Before ALS, I could allow myself forty-five minutes to get ready every morning. Eventually, it required more than two hours. I would still be late at times, because unpredictable mishaps would eat up my allotted time for preparation.

I would come home late. Then, I would work on my computer for another couple of hours. It wasn't possible to get to bed early. Getting ready for bed took longer, too. I was getting less sleep than I needed, and this was aggravating my symptoms, making my coordination worse. In turn, predictably, this was causing even greater inefficiency. I was sinking in a vicious cycle, but I could not escape my new reality.

In Florida, in the summer, it rains every afternoon, like clockwork. I didn't use to mind. I could carry my purse, my bags, files, while holding an umbrella, all at the same time. Now, I couldn't. When I eventually began walking with a cane, I could only hold an umbrella, if I was going to stay dry. Just walking to the building where I worked took much longer than it used to. Everyone was so nice. My legal assistant would meet me at my car and carry my file boxes into the office for me, but traveling to appointments was becoming a major challenge. During the rainy season, I often arrived at my destination soaked by rain. I couldn't dash from my car to the shelter of a lobby. As a lawyer, you are expected to look professional. How professional can you look, drenched to the bone?

Then, there was the falling. It didn't matter how much care that I was taking. I began to fall every once in a while, regardless. And with each fall, my fear of falling was increased. Eventually, I reached a point of severe anxiety. It was just so embarrassing. I remember one time in particular. I was walking to the courthouse. It was raining. I was juggling my purse, legal files, umbrella, and probably a few other things. I caught my heel on a grate in the sidewalk. I went flying forward. I couldn't even break my fall, because I was carrying so many things. Instead, I sacrificed myself. I appeared at trial with skin scraped off my hand, a baseball sized bump on my forehead, and drenched hair and suit. I hated it. How could I take on the world and win my case, when I couldn't even catch myself when I stumbled?

Once, when walking across uneven ground, I lost my balance. I fell on my face, and scraped the skin on my face. It stayed that way for quite some time, and covering the scrapes with makeup took a lot of time and effort. Another time, I was working late at my office. As I stood up quickly, I felt dizzy. I turned to pick something up, lost my balance and fell backwards. This resulted in a sore butt and low back, but no injuries, thank God. At this time, I was trying the ketogenic diet, which doesn't allow many carbs. It didn't help because it made me dizzy.

Most embarrassingly, I fell during a deposition. In a deposition, a lawyer asks a potential witness in a trial questions as part of discovery. The potential witness is called the deponent. There are always a lot of documents at a deposition. A lawyer uses the deposition to put the documents gathered during the discovery process in context. Since not every witness tells the truth voluntarily, a lawyer also uses the documents to prompt truthful answers from the deponent. While we were taking a break, I was standing at a large table reviewing documents that I would be using to pin the witness down on some facts important in the case. For no reason, I felt myself starting to fall backward. Thinking quickly, I grabbed onto a chair to steady myself. Unfortunately, this chair was on wheels. Instead of steadying me, the chair moved with me. I danced with the chair until the back of my head hit the wall and my body crashed to the floor. Thankfully, my assistant was the only one in the room, and she was so sweet. I was able to retain some dignity. She helped me up, but the fall caused significant bruising and a massive headache, but the show must go on. If the witness and his attorney had been there, I would have been mortified.

Another fall happened in my own bathroom at home. I felt myself starting to fall. I was determined not to fall. I dug my nails into the counter top. I fell backwards, anyway. Part of my fingernails tore away from my fingers, leaving my fingers bleeding and bruised, and still the back of my head fell right onto the base of the scale in the bathroom. I had another contusion and a severe headache. What's more, with every fall, I was losing faith that I could prevent myself from falling.

My own fear of falling, perhaps in combination with the disease ravaging my body, caused me such anxiety that my body would freeze. I would be standing there like a statue, unable to move at all. Whenever this happened, I would be stuck in the same place for several minutes. The more I struggled to move, the more panic would grip my mind. The more rigid my body would become. Only by consciously calming myself could I relax my muscles, allowing myself to walk again.

My fear of falling began to cause panic attacks. I had never had a single panic attack in my life before this time. I was accustomed to high-stress situations. I am a trial attorney. I always handled stress very well. I could manage the fear standing in front of a jury, a judge, my adversaries on the other side and possibly a hostile witness. I was calm under this type of pressure. Focused. Impervious. So, when I began having severe panic attacks, as a result of my fear of falling. I was disgusted. Pathetic. How pathetic. My heart would race. I could hear my heart pounding in my ears. I would feel a weight pressing down hard on my chest. My breathing would become rapid all because I couldn't control my own body!

I didn't want to tell anyone about these panic attacks. I had always been so self-sufficient. At one point in time, a panic attack came on as I was getting out of my car in a parking garage at work. I actually felt that I was going to suffocate and die. It was so bad that I called my husband, who drove to where I was parked and he was able to talk me through it, to help me calm down. I was not alone. I believe that it was the fear of falling while walking into work that caused the panic. It was just so mortifying to show up at work with scrapes and contusions. That was probably the most frightening and most embarrassing moment of my life. I had to admit the panic that I was feeling to someone else. I never needed support from anyone. From an emotional standpoint, I was a rock. I was the one providing emotional support to others. I did not need it, myself. I had always been in control. The idea of needing help, especially emotional help, was humiliating.

The most terrifying thing about ALS for me is that I can see everything it does to my body as it is happening. It's not a disease that allows you to feel and look fine, but then you find out it is spreading after getting an X-ray or MRI. PALS can see its effects hour by hour, day by day, and week by week. You can see and feel the disease progressing and spreading to other areas of your body that were healthy just yesterday. Believe me, it happens just that fast. I remember that it did for me after I was diagnosed and before I was on the Deanna Protocol®.

For example, I knew that the disease was in my left leg, so I would focus on my right leg that worked fine. I would rely more on that leg and think positively about that leg because it worked. One morning, I woke up and realized my right leg was twitching. Within a couple of weeks, the disease had spread to that leg and it was very hard to move that leg. Then, I tried to stay positive and focus on the fact that I still could use my arms and hands. One morning, I woke up and my left arm started to twitch. Within a couple of weeks, I had limited range of motion in that arm and it felt very weak. This is how it happened with every area of my body, my remaining good arm, my hands, my mouth, my voice, etc. Watching the spread of ALS weakening my body piece by piece and not being able to do anything about it is a horrific experience. It's frustrating. It's infuriating. It's humiliating. It's demoralizing.

For a while, I was scared to go to sleep at night because I knew there would always be a chance that I would wake up and find that ALS had spread to another part of my body. I would also get nervous anticipating and trying to predict where it would show up next. I never knew. It was always a waiting game and always a surprise. ALS is mental torture. More than most people realize, it takes a lot of effort to stay positive and to fight off psychological disorders that result from having ALS, such as depression, phobia, anxiety.

Many ALS patients have severe depression, and I completely understand. I am able to cope with my bouts of sadness without taking antidepressants. I have never been one to enjoy a pity party. So, I try to maintain a relentlessly positive attitude and give myself frequent pep talks every time I'm feeling down. Perhaps that's what has saved me.

After my diagnosis, my dad seemed to spend every

waking moment figuring out my disease and how to help me. I was grateful for his dedication, but I also felt guilty. His life was all of a sudden all about me. He had worked so hard for over thirty years in a stressful job with little sleep, and he finally had time to relax. I took that away from him and he didn't even seem to mind. I guess the saying is true; there is no love like a parent's love for his or her child. That was something I would not experience as a parent, but I felt and still feel very lucky to be on the receiving end of such love.

Before the Deanna Protocol®, my body was declining very rapidly. Of course, the fast pace of my disease worried me. Soon, I needed a cane to walk. Even with the cane, I walked very slowly. I couldn't carry anything without the worry of dropping it. I needed help with a lot of things because my hands were so shaky. I was still working as a partner at a law firm and I worked long hours. People I worked with knew I had a neurological condition, but nobody knew I had ALS, except the head partners, and I tried my best to cover it up. My reasoning was that, if my brain was fine, I should be able to work. I thought that being a good attorney had nothing to do with having an able body, so I was determined to keep working. Getting ready in the morning became like a rat race between me, my mom, and Don. When I arrived at my office, my assistant would carry things to and from my car for me. I had never depended much on other people, and it took some getting used to.

However, you'd be amazed at what people will say. Someone asked, "So, do you know what your nerve issue is yet?" I answered "Um, no. The doctors still have to do more tests. I'll be fine though." I smiled, hoping she would leave. Her answer was "Oh man, well I hope it's not ALS. If I had ALS, I would just end my own life. There's really no point to life when you get that type of diagnosis." I resented her comment. There is a point to life. Life is even more precious with *that type of diagnosis*. Of course, those close to me were supportive and tried to reassure me that I would be OK. I knew I had ALS and they didn't, at first. I was probably too serious, independent and private for my own good. I've had to learn how to laugh at myself. I've found that this is one of the best defenses against this disease.

One morning, I was walking to the court house with a cane while carrying my purse, a file and an umbrella. I was crossing the street in front of a line of cars that were stopped at a light in downtown morning rush hour. It was a windy day and, again my hands were full. Suddenly, a gust of wind blew my skirt up, not just a little, but all the way to my chin, exposing my underwear to everyone. I cursed the wind, but it just blew my hair in front of my eyes. I was panicking, trying to switch my purse to the hand holding the cane to use a free hand to recover some modesty. I was becoming frustrated and embarrassed with my clumsiness. Then, cars started honking, and I began to laugh. I just simply stopped caring and the whole situation became hilarious to me. No doubt, the people in those stopped cars, thought that I had escaped from the asylum. I remember thinking "Oh, damn! What underwear am I wearing today?" I couldn't remember. "I hope they're cute, at least!" I thought, chuckling.

Later, I'll talk about the roller coaster my dad and I rode together with all of the new supplements I tried, all of the dosages that had to be modified, and what the supplements did to me. Here though, I'll reveal what was happening in my mind because I think it's an important aspect of ALS to acknowledge. I switched my mental state from denial, to fear and sadness, to acceptance, determination and humor. Now, my mental state changed several times a week, and it was not a linear process. I would be crying and depressed one day, then laughing and telling friends and family about the clumsy things I had done the next day, hoping they would laugh with me.

I decided that my husband, Don, the love of my life, should get on with his life. I was sitting in bed and Don came in the room. "Babe", I tried to get his attention. "I need to talk to you." He sat down next to me "What's up?" "I need to talk to you and I don't want you to interrupt me," I said. He chuckled, "I know better than to interrupt a lawyer. Are you cross examining me? Do I need to have my own attorney present?" This made me laugh, but I was serious. "Seriously, we need to talk," I continued. "OK," Don said, getting down to business. "You know what ALS is, right? You know about everything it does to the body, the life expectancy, the care that patients with ALS need... day in and day out, the money that it costs? You looked it up?" I paused. Don answered, "Yes...what are you getting at?" I felt weak and my heart began to pound. I was frightened of the conversation I was starting. "OK, well I love you very much and we've already been through a lot with the baby and all; I appreciate your love and support so much, I really do...but you should leave me. I won't be mad. You're still young, you can find someone else. You don't have to deal with this. I want you to be happy." Don looked at me in disbelief. His words were, "Deanna, stop it; this is ridiculous."

I breathed deeply trying to prevent tears. My throat was closing up and I reminded myself of why I was having this conversation. Keep the conversation on track, Deanna. Don't get caught in the emotions. It is what it is. I thought. Then I reassured myself that I was right to bring this up. He shouldn't have to feel trapped and miserable being married to a dying nonfunctional wife and waiting on me hand and foot. "Leave. Leave while you can. Don't feel obligated to stay."

Don interrupted me. "Stop it. Stop insulting me and our marriage. I'm aware of the prognosis. However, I know this disease will not kill you. I just know. I have a feeling. I can't explain it. In terms of you being disabled; I'm prepared for it all. I'm not going anywhere, and you're offending me by saying I should..." His eyes looked steadily at me, his face was serious, and his voice had a sweet understanding tone to it...completely opposite of mine at this moment.

I was getting frustrated. "It's not even about me being disabled. Anything we had, anything we were...it's all going to be gone! Forget the former Don and Deanna. The relationship that existed is going away." My throat tightened again and my eyes began to burn. I hugged my pillow. I began to cry and hugged my pillow closely. He put his arm on my shoulder. I moved away from him and let his arm fall onto the bed. "You didn't sign up for this. This marriage will consist of you giving me everything and me taking everything from you, but giving nothing back!"

Don smiled, "I did sign up for this. This is exactly what I signed up for. This is what marriage is about. It's not all roses and parties." "You think I haven't thought about this?" He asked. "You think I'm pretending it's not real?" He continued. "I have thought about it, day and night. I've thought about what you could be like if we don't find a way to stop this disease and what it will be like to watch ALS take over you and our lives. I've thought about that every second, so stop reminding me." Then, he asked, "Do you know what I have not thought about?" He paused, "Leaving you. Not once has that thought crossed my mind and it never will. You can accept it or you can fight it, but either way, I'll be here, so you might as well stop fighting."

I lost it at this point. My heart rate began to slow down, my hands stopped shaking, my eyes welled up in tears, and I began to sob uncontrollably. "But...it's better...for you to leave...you won't be happy." I replied. "Babe, being your husband makes me happy. I will be one hundred times happier as the husband of Deanna with ALS than I would be with any other woman on earth who is perfectly healthy."

"You should have a choice..." I continued robotically, between sobs, not willing to give up, but Don wasn't having it. "I choose you. I didn't just make this choice on our wedding day. I make this choice every single day. I'll continue making this same choice every day for the rest of our lives. I choose you."

"K," was all I could utter, not even the O would come out. "Wait! Did I just actually win an argument with you? That'd be a yes." Don said, removing one arm from my back, patted himself on the shoulder, and gave me a smug grin. I just wrapped my arms around him again while I laughed and sobbed into his chest simultaneously for a good fifteen minutes. He kept cracking jokes to make me laugh, none of which I can remember. He rubbed my head, kissed me, and continued to tell me all of the reasons why he loved me. None of those reasons he cited had anything to do with me having a voice or a functioning body. They had everything to do with my mind and my heart, which I knew would stay intact.

I was always told that I will know when I've met "the one" when I can say to myself without any reservations that I love him much more than I love myself and he loves me much more than he loves himself. This moment reminded me that I chose the right husband. If we didn't have this type of love, I wouldn't have tried to convince him to leave, and he would have already left. This is something that all couples afflicted with ALS deal with, the question of whether the healthy spouse is willing and able to stick around when things get ugly. Unfortunately, many ALS patients are abandoned by their spouses, even those who have no other family to support them. They're left completely alone. I have heard more of these stories than I can stomach. ALS is not for the faint hearted.

I have had a few similar conversations with Don, where I tried to convince him that it was OK to leave. These were shorter and less dramatic, and I was prepared to lose him. These conversations usually occurred while I was having a sad day and feeling sorry for both him and myself. We don't have these conversations anymore.

My husband is my rock supporting me and coming to my rescue whenever I need him most. My dad was about to come to my rescue, also.

Chapter Eight

Dr. Tedone's Research

Sometimes, all you have to hang onto is a thread. For me, in this situation, the thread was toxins. I began to research ways to test toxins and ways to remove toxins from the body. Deanna had received Dr. Carter's report a few days after returning from seeing The Undertaker, and she called me. I picked up the phone and listened.

"Dad, you'll never believe what Dr. Carter said in her report."

"What's that?" I was curious.

Deanna read from the report, "Mrs. Tedone-Gage definitely has ALS, although I am not going to reveal this information at this time. She is here with her father and I will reveal her true diagnosis when she returns with her husband."

"She knew the whole time?" I questioned, surprised to hear this for the first time.

"Yup" Deanna answered. "And she never told me I had ALS when I went back with Don either. She just told me to come back in a few months so she could evaluate me."

Who would do a thing like that, I thought? It is one thing if she's not ready to make a diagnosis, but it's quite another to make the diagnosis and hide it from a person. Nevertheless, I asked Deanna to call Dr. Carter and try to convince her to test her for strontium. My research had convinced me that it was the strontium in the Chinese drywall that caused the dwarfed, deformed fetus. I wondered if it was strontium that triggered Deanna's ALS.

Surprisingly, Deanna was actually able to convince her. We received the report back and the results showed very low levels of strontium in her blood. I wasn't surprised or disappointed. Now, I knew that the strontium from the Chinese drywall was fixed in Deanna's tissues, but how can Deanna get rid of it. If she could get rid of the toxins, would she be well?

During the course of my research, I read about a technique called chelation, a process by which toxins can be removed from the body. I thought that this might be the answer. Deanna tried chelation for some time and I was hopeful that it would work, but it didn't. Perhaps, toxins were being removed from her body by chelation, but the chelation did not slow or stop the progression of her ALS. Chelation made no difference. Worse, yet, I was to learn from a brilliant toxicologist that chelation, if anything, may have made Deanna's disease progress faster by putting more of the toxins back in Deanna's circulatory system. I regret my decision to try chelation, and I strongly recommend that PALS not try it.

I watched my daughter's health deteriorate week after week. She was experiencing twitching in her legs and arms, her balance issues were becoming worse, and she was walking very slowly. Eventually, her range of motion was very limited, and she became so spastic that she could not carry a water glass without spilling it. Most objects that she picked up, she would drop. By this time, she was walking very slowly with a strong left to right sway. She was also having trouble turning over in bed.

My first attempt didn't work. I had failed, utterly, to even slow down the progression of Deanna's disease. I needed something else. I was going to help my daughter. There was a solution and all I had to do was find it. Perseverance, challenge the status quo, do what is necessary, even if unconventional. Deanna knew that the chelation didn't stop the disease and she was scared as she watched the disease attack her body piece by piece. "Dad," I remember her saying. "I'm getting worse. I know it. I don't know what to do."

"I promise you that this is not the end. I will find something else to try to attack it." She did not reveal the slightest bit of doubt. She nodded and said, "Whatever I need to do, and I'm on board." Deanna showed such courage. This was only the beginning of our journey and only the start of Deanna's incredible display of courage. This girl was fearless. Just as she had been, always.

During this time, I met with and spoke to a variety of neurologists and toxicologists about toxins and the link to ALS. The neurologists would tell me "Well, I'm not a toxicologist." The toxicologists would tell me "Well, I'm not a neurologist." The neurologists and toxicologists I called were world renowned in their fields and worked at prestigious institutions, yet none of them had answers and none seemed to have interest in collaborating with each other to try to tackle ALS. To me, this is shocking. If toxicologists know that toxins cause ALS, how can you let this go? If neurologists don't know if toxins cause ALS, how can you let this go?

I felt alone. My colleagues seemed to think I was crazy for even attempting to slow or stop the progression of ALS. It felt like the entire neurology community had accepted the fact that ALS has no cure or treatment and the fact that I questioned this made me some sort of radical in their eyes. This would not stop me. I had dedicated my life to finding a treatment for ALS, something that could slow or stop the progression of the disease.

But was this just arrogance? How could one conceivably think that they could solve a problem that has been around for two-hundred or more years and that so many intelligent people have been working on, spending billions of dollars a year to solve and yet haven't been able to? Where does that kind of hubris come from? No, it is not hubris. My life taught me that only by perseverance can the impossible become possible. It isn't hubris to love your daughter more than your own life. It isn't hubris to hope beyond hope for a breakthrough. A breakthrough was coming, or I would die trying.

Progress is painstakingly slow when trying to understand a disease as difficult as ALS. Trial and error, mostly error, won't make progress. This disease progresses so rapidly. I needed answers. I wanted them yesterday, but nothing seemed to work. Drugs in clinical trials failed, routinely. Promising research hit dead ends. We need a breakthrough, and we needed it soon. I could see my daughter slipping away, every day, to this awful disease.

Chapter Nine

Deanna's Courage

My dad kept up a steady pace of research and a steady stream of remedies, which were all safe for humans. I knew what would happen if I did nothing, and my dad was careful to monitor my condition and to terminate anything that made me worse. Chelation therapy didn't work. I tried the ketogenic diet and ketone boosting supplements with no result. Many things didn't work. Also, even if regarded as safe, there were side effects. With everything that I was trying, each day was a surprise. I never knew how I would feel when I woke up or even immediately after taking some new supplement. It might affect my energy levels or coordination and some things didn't sit right in my stomach. My stomach has been through a lot.

The very worst substance for my stomach, by far, was a proprietary substance that I took, which was supposed to boost my ketone levels. It was a thick oil-like liquid that I had to drink. The liquid had an oil-like consistency and tasted how I would imagine toxic chemical sludge would taste. I nicknamed it "Jet Fuel." The minute the liquid touched my lips, I would feel my gag reflex and nausea in my stomach. After swallowing it down, it would coat my entire mouth and throat. The lingering taste would make the nausea worse.

I soon learned to coat my mouth with something good immediately after drinking this. My food of choice was chocolate and man, did I shove it in my mouth quickly! That melting chocolate was an angel to me. After swallowing the liquid, my nausea became worse and I felt pains in my stomach for hours after taking it. I began to eat substantial meals before taking it, which prevented me from throwing up, but did not completely alleviate stomach pain. My sister was curious about the taste, so she dipped the tip of her finger in my glass one day and briefly touched her finger to her tongue. Her eyes immediately began to tear up. You get the idea of the type of taste I was dealing with.

I drank this liquid multiple times a day for a few months. The results were disappointing. Not only was I nauseous, but also my stomach bloated to the point that I looked pregnant. My condition continued to worsen over time. In addition to the Jet Fuel, I had to prick my finger with a blood-testing implement to check for ketone bodies several times a day and record my ketone levels all day to see whether they were high enough for the treatment to be effective. This lasted for a few weeks and my fingers were bruised and sore from constantly being pricked. I had to go through this regimen merely to rule out a treatment that didn't work, but I am glad I did. I knew that my dad was leaving no stone unturned in searching for a treatment for ALS. It was much better than the alternative offered by neurologists, to sit back and wait for ALS to kill me.

I tried a stem cell stimulating substance in an attempt to regenerate the motor neurons that were dying in my body. This substance did not bother my stomach, but it had other side effects. When I received an injection, I would notice a change in my body within hours. I felt groggy. Moving my arms and legs was a chore, so walking was tough. I walked with a cane, but after the injection, I would need a cane on one side and a person on the other side to link arms with me so I wouldn't fall. It didn't work.

Then I tried another drug, and after three injections, my arm had blown up to twice its normal size. I also couldn't see very well. I remember stumbling into my bathroom and being shocked when I looked in the mirror. My face was red, my lips puffed out like collagen injections gone wrong, and each of my eyes was a small slit in between two tiny red moon shaped pillows, which used to be my eyelids. I looked down and my hands, feet, and legs were swollen too. It took several days for the swelling to go down completely. Needless to say, that drug was out.

Most treatments that we tried tasted foul and hurt my stomach. I became used to the discomfort. I won't go through every failure, but my dad and I went through quite the struggle in trying to find a treatment for ALS. He researched all day and into the night and always seemed to come up with something new to investigate or to try on me. He was very careful and never tried anything blindly. He always researched side effects of the different substances. He made sure they were safe to use on humans. He would read every study he could get his hands on, and questioned the rationale behind using each treatment for ALS. Those treatments that passed his tests, I would try.

This was an emotional roller coaster for me, filled with hope and disappointment. I was filled with hope every time I heard of a new treatment and was crushed every time a treatment didn't work. It was exhausting and I guess it would have been less of a rollercoaster for me if I refrained from having hope until I saw results. However, I couldn't help but have hope whenever my dad told me about something new he was planning to try. Somehow, I felt that I needed that hope. That hope gave me something to focus on aside from my death sentence. It helped me fight to stay alive, despite the fact that my body was becoming weaker. As long as there was something out there that might work, I could reasonably say to myself Deanna, you have to survive. What if this next treatment works for you? If you give up on yourself now, you will never benefit from it.

My dad never once gave up on me. After everything he tried in the earlier stages failed, he still kept at it. I kept waiting for the day that he would lose steam. After all, there are only so many failed treatments one man can try before saying "enough is enough." Not my dad. He never loses steam. He never seemed discouraged. Every failure was a success in a way, because it made way for something new to try. Knowing that he was working so hard at finding a way to treat ALS removed some of the stress from my mind. Any time I would become anxious, I would think to myself, "Don't worry. Dad's got this." Even when giving up makes complete logical sense, even when all of his colleagues tell him it's a lost cause, giving up just isn't in his DNA.

Chapter Ten

Dr. Tedone's Breakthrough

The most rewarding successes start in failure. In the early days, immediately following Deanna's diagnosis, we tried a host of different substances and none proved successful. Deanna was so courageous and nothing that I was trying was having any positive effects. There were no encouraging signs that anything would work.

On one of our visits at a prestigious institution, I asked the neurologist if it were his mother or daughter what he would prescribe for her. He said Rocephin®. I researched Rocephin® and found out that it was in phase 2 clinical trials and had applied for phase 3 approval. Rocephin® is an antibiotic readily available. There were several reports from PALS on the ALS blogs on the internet, who were on Rocephin® all were negative. The treatment was very expensive and required an intravenous infusion twice a day. Then, I learned that it had not been accepted for phase 3. This was obviously not a choice for my daughter.

While sitting in my office one day, as I was thinking about Rocephin®, the following questions occurred to me. Why did anyone ever try Rocephin® for treating ALS? Why would scientists have ever suspected that Rocephin® might be effective? I started to do some research to find out the answer to my questions, and the answer would eventually lead to a breakthrough.

The National Institute of Health (NIH) funded a multi-institutional study to find something that could break glutamate down in ALS patients.[11] In response to the NIH, scientists screened thousands of substances to determine if any of them could break down glutamate. They found Rocephin®. High-throughput screening is a type of brute force trial and error screening, which is a favorite of big pharmaceutical companies that have the resources to screen, in parallel, thousands of substances to identify a few candidates that will be further developed as drugs. In this case, there was not enough evidence that it could help Deanna.

However, the fact that the National Institute of Health was studying glutamate as an essential factor in the ALS equation got me thinking. If glutamate is important in ALS, why is it important? It gave me a place to start, when toxins provided me nothing. Some researchers believe that excess glutamate causes glutamate excitotoxicity, which contributes to neuron cell death perhaps spreading the disease from cell to cell.[12]

Excess glutamate can cause abnormal sodium and

---

11   Heemskerk, J., Tobin, A.J., and Bain, L.J. (2002). Teaching old drugs new tricks. *Trends in Neurosciences, 25*(10), 494–496. DOI: http://dx.doi.org/10.1016/S0166-2236(02)02236-1.

12   Redler R.L., & Dokholyan, N.V. (2012). The complex molecular biology of amyotrophic lateral sclerosis (ALS). *Prog Mol Biol Transl Sci. 107*, 215–262. http://www.ncbi.nlm.nih.gov/pmc/articles/PMC3605887.

potassium to flow into and out of the cells, which can cause excessive fluid to build up in the nerve cells. I picture these cells as water balloons that burst, releasing their contents into the extracellular fluid. I didn't need to know how glutamate damages cells in order to treat the disease. If I could find a way to break down glutamate in the body, this could be an effective way of treating ALS and other neurodegenerative diseases. I was curious to see how the body's own natural enzymes break down glutamate. Glutamate dehydrogenase (GDH) and glutamate decarboxylase (GAD) metabolize glutamate in the body in a process called the Krebs cycle. The Krebs cycle is a complex cycle that provides energy to the cells and without energy, the cells die.

I spoke with a variety of labs to see if they could compound GDH and GAD. I found out that, in the best case scenario, if GDH could be compounded, it would cost $1,000 per gram. Unfortunately, the enzyme isn't stable, either, and even intravenous or intramuscular injections would probably not effectively deliver enough GDH to the neurons to do much good.

I don't get discouraged easily. If I can't get GDH to the cells, then I had to look at the precursors to GDH and GAD. Could I get these into the body and let the body produce the GDH and GAD? Unfortunately, I found that the precursor to GDH and GAD enzymes are genes. There is very little publicly available literature on these genes. I was venturing in a direction that was practically untouched by science and beyond my understanding, so I couldn't continue in that direction. Since neither I nor the NIH could provide a substance that breaks down glutamate effectively, I decided that my time was best spent looking elsewhere. But where?

I decided to look at the other end of the cycle. I started investigating the substances derived from glutamate. I reasoned that if the body can't break down glutamate, then, perhaps, the cells lack whatever substances are being produced in the breakdown of glutamate. I found that when GDH and GAD break down glutamate, alpha-Ketoglutarate (AKG) and gamma-amino butyric acid (GABA) are produced. If PALS lack the enzymes to break down glutamate, it follows that PALS lack AKG and GABA in their bodies. Both AKG and GABA are available on the market for humans and are considered safe for human consumption.

I decided to try GABA on Deanna. Deanna and I went to a neurologist at an esteemed institution, who I will not identify here. I asked him what I could use to control Deanna's spasticity and rigidity. He suggested the prescription drug Baclofen®. I researched this comparatively expensive drug and found out that it is GABA with an alteration to allow it to pass the blood brain barrier (BBB). I started giving Deanna GABA, which is not particularly expensive, and the results were encouraging. For the first time in several months, she could carry a glass of water without shaking and spilling it. So, enough of the GABA was getting to where it needs to be, without the expensive alteration incorporated into the prescription drug. Sometimes, I wonder if big pharma comes out with proprietary products just to keep the competition at bay.

The next substance to try was AKG. AKG is an acid and can be very hard on the stomach. Instead, I gave Deanna arginine alpha-Ketoglutarate (AAKG), a salt and a dietary supplement, which is available for human consumption. Body builders use AAKG to recover from heavy exercise and to help them build muscle. Arginine is an alpha-amino acid that is already present in the body. So, it was unlikely to cause any harm, and makes AKG more tolerable for the digestive system. Arginine might even be beneficial, but at the time, I did not know if arginine could help Deanna.

I gave Deanna AAKG for a couple of months, building up the dosing slowly. Side effects for AAKG can include water retention, stomach upset and diarrhea. So, some caution is necessary. Ramping up AAKG lets you know how much can be tolerated and how much is needed for a particular person. Deanna noticed her fasciculations and twitching subsided and she was also able to turn over in bed normally without having to be on her knees. These signs of improvement were so remarkable, because Deanna's health had been deteriorating daily before adding GABA and AAKG to her diet.

Remarkably, when Deanna ran out of AAKG after a couple of months, only a day after stopping the AAKG, she went from walking with a cane to barely being able to walk at all. There was a marked increase in twitching and fasciculations in the muscles. She became worse every day that she went without the AAKG. Then, when Deanna resumed AAKG, these symptoms went away, again. This was proof enough for me to know that AKG and GABA are important dietary supplements lacking in PALS. At the time, I thought that the excess glutamate was caused by a breakdown in the body's ability to create the enzymes to further process glutamate. I know now that glutamate is not in excess but just displaced out of the cell so it cannot be metabolized to produce AKG and GABA. Without AKG and GABA, Deanna's symptoms became worse. With AAKG and GABA, Deanna's symptoms improved.

Finally, some success! Everyone else was looking for drugs to get rid of excess glutamate, but I looked at what was missing if the body was not metabolizing glutamate properly. This was the genesis of the Deanna Protocol®. We still had much work to do. How much AAKG and GABA are needed? When should it be administered? How can it be administered? Is there anything that can be done to reverse the damage already done to PALS?

Next, I looked at the metabolic process relating to AKG. Coenzymes CoQ10 and NADH are required in the metabolic process in which AKG is involved. So, I added coenzymes CoQ10 and NADH to the Deanna Protocol®. Actually, I added a more potent form of CoQ10, called Ubiquinol®. NADH is not well absorbed in the stomach. It can be administered in other ways, but I decided to try precursors of NADH, niacin and 5-hydroxytryptophane. These seemed to help, but the main ingredients, AAKG and GABA had the most dramatic impact on my daughter's symptoms. Caution must be taken with niacin, because it is known to be toxic to cells and the liver if taken in excess.

After starting the Deanna Protocol®, Deanna's strength started returning in some areas and her coordination is improving, overall. In other areas of her body, Deanna has not gained any strength and coordination, but at least the progression of the disease appears to have stopped.

As you might expect, I told a few people of my daughter's success with the AAKG and GABA. I am sure that I must have told everyone who had the patience to listen. Thank you all. Your kindness and patience is appreciated. Some of the people that I told spread the word to others. One of the earliest success stories that came back to me was actually from an individual who treated his wife with AAKG. His wife had Alzheimer's and was completely bed ridden in a vegetative state. She did not recognize her own children or her husband, could not remember who she was, and could not hold a conversation. After giving her the AAKG for a little over a week, her husband began to notice a difference in her. After taking the AAKG for a few months, the results were astonishing. He told me that his wife was now standing, remembered him and her children, speaking, holding conversations, watching TV, and she had even remembered her wedding anniversary!

I received other accounts of ALS patients taking AAKG and being able to walk again after spending a couple of months in a wheel chair. I received reports of ALS patients being able to chew solid food again after months of being restricted to liquid and reports of them being able to speak more clearly. This was very encouraging anecdotal evidence but I knew we needed more to convince neurologists to try the Deanna Protocol® with their PALS, even though it makes intuitive sense.

Why are AKG and GABA so important to the body? AKG is a ketone that helps the body's energy cycle run efficiently. GABA is an inhibitory neurotransmitter, which relaxes the muscles. It balances the excitatory neurotransmitters, which can cause muscles to become spastic (i.e. tense and rigid) in PALS. When the body has more excitatory neurotransmitters (e.g. glutamate) than inhibitory neurotransmitters (i.e. GABA), the imbalance causes spasticity, which make it extremely difficult for people with neurodegenerative diseases to control their own muscles. Therefore, it is important that PALS have enough GABA to relax the muscles. My view has changed in relation to what causes the abnormal muscle tone. Neuro scientists initially attributed the excitotoxicity to excess glutamate, we now know the glutamate is not in excess just displaced out of the cell.

Exercise is important to retain muscle mass. I began to wonder about exercise and how it would affect Deanna's ALS. Of course, every single neurologist I spoke to said it would be a bad idea for Deanna to exercise. Their advice was based on the observation that exercise in PALS caused more rapid muscle wasting than not exercising. This seemed counter intuitive to me, that exercise would cause muscles to atrophy more quickly than lack of exercise. It supports the idea that the cells in PALS lack energy. However, the solution is not to stop exercising, but when exercising, it is necessary to supply more energy to the cells. Deanna does this by taking more AAKG before and while she exercises.

I started Deanna on an exercise regimen which, at first, concentrated on her legs, and then, extended to other areas of her body. More will be explained about the exercise regimen later, but the overall result was that her strength improved in many areas.

As a note, the response of increased muscle symptoms upon stopping AAKG, only to have the muscle symptoms decline when AAKG is resumed, has been repeated many times by PALS, who have reported this to us through our website www.winningthefight.org. If you are not taking enough AKG, you will notice the following muscle symptoms: fasciculation and twitching. If you are taking enough AKG, these symptoms decline. As with many metabolic processes, the right amount of AKG depends on an individual's body, diet and lifestyle. Deanna notices that she needs more when she exercises. So, we gauge the required dose of AAKG by the presence or absence of muscle symptoms. If muscle symptoms persist, more AAKG is needed. There is a limit. Eventually, the water retention and stomach upset side effects caused by taking too much AAKG limits the amount that can be taken. Deanna has been fortunate, because she tolerates AAKG well.

Likewise, for GABA, which controls spasticity (i.e. a jerking motion of the limbs), also rigidity, tremors and cramps. These symptoms of spasticity indicate that more GABA is needed. This can be monitored by PALS, and more can be taken as necessary.

Chapter Eleven

Deanna's Prognosis

I am not free of ALS. Even with the Deanna Protocol®, life is a constant challenge, but it's a challenge that I'm happy to be around to tackle. My symptoms have stopped progressing rapidly. Some of them have reversed. I can do things that I could not do. My strength is coming back to me. I feel blessed to have such a loving family and my husband, Don, by my side. The Deanna Protocol® has made a tremendous difference in my life, and I am able to fight back against ALS, finally.

I am working to build strength in my muscles that had atrophied prior to finding the Deanna Protocol®. It still takes time to get ready for the day and to get ready for bed at night, but I can still do it. I want PALS to know about the Deanna Protocol® before it is too late, before they have to suffer what I have suffered. The Deanna Protocol® delays the disease. Maybe it could prevent the disease from progressing to the point that mine has, if started earlier.

The Deanna Protocol® won't help everyone. Those with later stage ALS can benefit from increased energy and more comfort. However, we don't know if it will prolong life because as you will read later on, the Deanna Protocol® gives nerve and muscle cells energy, and in the later stages, it does not stop the progression, entirely. We don't know why, but we are trying to find out.

I warn PALS that not all dietary supplements are equal. There are forums on www.winningthefight.org to share information on brands that are reputable. In addition, being consistent with the Deanna Protocol® is very important along with cataloging your symptoms before taking the Deanna Protocol® and after. If you are like me, it will take some time to get the balance of exercise and supplements right because as you deplete your energy, you will need to replenish it by taking more than the suggested doses. I continue to experiment on myself, adjusting levels of nutritional substances.

I also can't emphasize enough how important exercise is in a battle with ALS, and how important it is to surround yourself with trained professionals who are on the same page as you. I'm fortunate to have an amazing team consisting of a personal trainer, a physical therapist, hand therapist and speech therapist all of whom are focused on improving my function. This is important because so many professionals treat people with ALS like a foregone conclusion i.e. your demise is imminent, and there's nothing you can do. To avoid professionals like this, you must interview them because you are essentially hiring them for an extremely important job, and if you're not on the same page with the same goals of maintaining function and or improving, you're wasting your time.

While the Deanna Protocol® gives you tools to physically fight ALS, your mental attitude is a key tool in fighting ALS too. ALS as a diagnosis is entangled in negativity, and as you can tell from my story, initially, I got sucked into the dark hole of negativity. It wasn't until I was told there's nothing you can do for the fourth time that I finally got angry and said "watch me!" This was even before my dad came up with the Deanna Protocol®. I firmly believe that a positive attitude will take you far in your fight. You will still get sad and frustrated for various reasons, but I think you'll notice those moments will be few and won't last long. You also need humor and to be able to laugh at yourself.

I'm not scared. I have hope, and my dad has not stopped. He is continuing to research therapies that can reverse the damage caused by the loss of motor neurons caused by ALS. There is promising research out of Israel that indicates that ALS can be beaten. My dad wants to start a clinical trial incorporating the Deanna Protocol® with a substance that removes glutamate. He believes that this will be the next phase and hopes that more of the symptoms can be reversed. He thinks that decreasing the levels of glutamate in the blood could stop the spreading of ALS to other muscle groups.

I don't understand neurologists' refusal to accept the Deanna Protocol®, including my own neurologist. PALS need these supplements to prevent rapid degeneration of their motor neurons and muscles. I am not an isolated case. Many PALS have been helped through word of mouth and the efforts of Winning the Fight, Inc. on its website: www.winningthefight.org.

We have not given up, and we are going to find a cure for ALS. Then, we are going to find a cure for other neurodegenerative diseases. Join our cause. Go to www.winningthefight.org. You can make a difference in PALS lives. Together, we will fight neurodegenerative disease, and we will win the fight.

Chapter Twelve

Dr. Tedone's Call to Action

I want every patient with ALS (PALS) to know about the Deanna Protocol®, preferably, even before a diagnosis is confirmed. Nutritional support of PALS is essential, because, fundamentally, ALS is a degenerative metabolic disease. Cells starve when the metabolic process is interrupted. But there is now hope. The dietary supplements combined in the Deanna Protocol®, exercise and massage are not difficult to obtain and are comparatively inexpensive. However our foundation, Winning the Fight, Inc., www.winningthefight.org, is encouraging manufacturers and distributors to make these dietary supplements even less expensive, more convenient and more palatable for PALS.

The pace of change is ever increasing. Even while writing, editing and preparing this book for publication, new research results and discoveries are occurring. We continue to improve the Deanna Protocol® for PALS and have realized that many patients with other neurodegenerative diseases could benefit from nutritional supplementation just like PALS. All neurodegenerative diseases, including ALS, have a metabolic component. It is my belief, confirmed by sponsored research, that the initial focus for patients should be to keep the patient's cells alive.

Otherwise, cells starved of energy die and probably lead to a cascading death of neighboring cells. This can lead to other complications, such as autoimmune disorders. Anecdotal evidence, reports from PALS on the Deanna Protocol® and recently published results in a study using ALS mice sponsored by Winning the Fight, Inc. are encouraging. Please go to our website: www.winningthefight.org for the latest information.

Drs. Teichberg and Ruban at the Weizmann Institute in Israel have been studying cell death in ALS. Drs. Teichberg and Ruban's focus is on documenting how the disease spreads in the body. When cells die, glutamate is released and this poisons nearby cells. This causes neighboring cells to die and leads to a devastating cascade effect. Other research confirms that toxic levels of extracellular glutamate kill human nerve cells. This process or a similar process might occur in other situations, such as Alzheimer's, Parkinson's, Multiple Sclerosis, tumors, traumatic brain injuries possibly including concussions and stroke.

Dr. Teichberg is deceased, but both Dr. Ruban and Dr. Tedone believe that these neurological diseases and those caused by trauma should be treated by preventing further cell death utilizing the Deanna Protocol® to support cell metabolism and neutralizing glutamate that is outside the cell with glutamate oxaloacetate transaminase (GOT). According to Dr. Ruban, preclinical studies have already been completed documenting a positive effect from neutralizing glutamate in ALS mice using GOT. It is our hope that clinical trials will soon be underway to document the benefit of neutralizing and removing excess glutamate with GOT. GOT is believed to be more stable than oxaloacetate in the body. We would like to include the Deanna Protocol® with GOT to determine if there is a synergistic effect. We hope that the DP + GOT would be even more effective than the DP alone.

Those pursuing a metabolic approach to these diseases are in the minority. The major portion of research has been done using a single drug to cure or treat these diseases. None of these pursuits have worked and, as a result, billions of dollars have been spent on this approach while thousands of patients are dying. You should understand what a disaster this is for patients, but why is it so difficult to change the direction of research?

It is so important for patients that we move the discussion forward to truly understand the mechanisms, genetic and environmental, which cause the onset and progression of neurodegenerative diseases, stroke, traumatic brain injury and autism. Until we do, metabolic dietary supplementation such as the Deanna Protocol® is the only effective therapy for PALS.

PART TWO

A Call to Action

Chapter Thirteen

Diagnosis

One of the most frustrating aspects of ALS is that it is so hard to diagnose. Some patients who have been diagnosed by a neurologist with ALS actually have other conditions that might be treated, if only the correct diagnosis was made. The most likely misdiagnosis of ALS is for those patients who suffer from Lyme disease. The authors warn clinicians that Lyme disease patients have more muscle pain than do patients with ALS. If patients present with muscle pain, then continue to look for Lyme disease, even if the first few tests come back negative. Another distinguishing clinical feature of Lyme disease is it is cyclical corresponding to the life cycle of the pathogen. When a virus or bacteria is in a dormant phase the symptoms subside. However, when the pathogen breaks out it causes an acute inflammatory reaction which is very painful. I have been asked why ALS is non painful since inflammation is also present. My thinking is that the inflammation in ALS is caused by ROS [reactive oxygen species] or free radicals which do not cause an acute response that bacteria causes; but rather a sub-acute or chronic infection that causes less swelling and hence less pain. Some PALS, who started the DP reported that their symptoms disappeared. We thought we had a miracle treatment. Then their pain and the symptoms returned—we knew those PALS did not have ALS. For example, the authors believe that about 20 patients diagnosed with ALS, registered on our web site actually had Lyme disease. Regardless, the Deanna Protocol® seems to provide some relief even to these patients, but misdiagnosing Lyme disease as ALS could prevent other antibiotic treatments from being used that could reverse the symptoms of patients suffering from Lyme disease and if administered early enough cure them.

A negative western blot test is insufficient to indicate the absence of Lyme disease. Further antibody tests are usually required at specific intervals in order to rule out Lyme disease. Clinically, intractable pain is often an indicator that the patient has Lyme disease and not ALS, but still, errors occur. However, waiting until Lyme disease can be ruled out to begin the Deanna Protocol® causes irreversible damage to PALS. So, my advice to clinicians is to start all patients with neurological deficits on the Deanna Protocol®. If the root cause is Lyme disease no harm will be done by giving the patient nutritional supplementation. If the patient has ALS, you could be saving his or her life.[13]

In 2002, five doctors published a scientific article that concluded that PALS were more likely to be slim or had once been serious athletes. For example, many people who died of ALS were athletes. Lou Gehrig, from which ALS gets its informal name, was a baseball player. Ezzard

---

13   http://www.borelioza.org/materialy_lyme/burrascano_10.2008.pdf.

Charles was a heavyweight-boxer. Catfish Hunter was a baseball player. The list of famous athletes in many different sports is too long to provide here. There appears to be a link between ALS and athleticism.[14] Deanna was thin and athletic before being diagnosed with ALS. These authors believe that ALS is a metabolic disorder, and the metabolism of athletes is somehow associated with the disease. The abstract claims: "Several famous athletes have been affected by ALS, and some epidemiologic studies have indicated that vigorous physical activity (heavy labor or athletics) is a risk factor for the disease." In a case-control study of 279 patients with motor neuron diseases and 152 with other neurologic diseases, the authors found that subjects with motor neuron diseases were more likely than controls to report they had always been slim or they had been varsity athletes. In the years before and following this study, several genetic factors have been tied to ALS, but no genetic disorder is responsible for more than 10% of PALS.[15]

The authors do not pretend that claiming that ALS is a metabolic disorder is not a controversial position, but we do ask you to consider the evidence before ruling out the role that metabolism plays in ALS. The efficacy of the

14   Scarmeas, N., Shih, T., Stern, Y., Ottman, R., Rowland, L. P. (2002). Premorbid Weight, Body Mass, and Varsity Athletics in ALS. *Neurology*, 59.5, 773–775. http://www.neurology.org/content/59/5/773.

15   In 2011, noncoding repeat expansions in C9ORF72 were found to be a major cause of ALS and front temporal dementia. C9orf72 (chromosome 9 open reading frame 72) is a protein which in humans is encoded by the gene C9orf72.

Deanna Protocol® is fully supported by all of the available research, and there are no studies known to the authors that bring into question the testimonials of so many PALS that have benefited from it.

The difficulty in confirming a diagnosis should not be a reason to dismiss the startling results reported in this Part Two of the Deanna Protocol®. Review the science with an open mind, and then, if you are convinced, help us to get the word out to PALS and to improve the Deanna Protocol®.

Chapter Fourteen

Overview

First, there is the science. If a lack of glutamate metabolism results in a lack of AKG and GABA, then PALS cells are short AKG and GABA, the metabolites of glutamate. The evidence for this mechanism will be presented later.

Then, there is Deanna's first person account contained in Part One of this book. The Deanna Protocol® stopped her hand tremors, spasticity, crushing fatigue and atrophy. There is the relapse when Deanna stopped taking AAKG and rebound when she restarted AAKG. There is the marked reduction in hand tremors when taking GABA. Deanna's ability to carry a glass, without dropping or spilling its contents, when she could not previously, is a sign of her improvement. There are Deanna's observations that her body needs more AAKG when exercising than when at rest. All of this evidence points to a condition that benefits from metabolic therapy, with improved muscle mass and strength from the combination of supplements, non-fatiguing exercise and massage with coconut oil, which are recommended in the Deanna Protocol® program.

Then, there are the ALSFRS scores of PALS.[16] The self-reported results of PALS indicate that the substances

16   See Appendix A the ALSFRS Scores.

provided by the Deanna Protocol® are helping PALS, whether correctly diagnosed or misdiagnosed. This is encouraging, even if a substantial number of PALS are mis-diagnosed. It is even more encouraging, when you consider that it is likely that many of the PALS reporting are trying to comply with recommendations without the active support of their clinical neurologist. According to skeptics, a synergistic combination of dietary supplements that support good metabolic health in motor neurons should have NO positive results in PALS. The self-reported observations from PALS undermine the skeptics' viewpoint.

There is the study in SOD1-G93A mice.[17] It cannot be denied. The DP® made a statistically significant difference in longevity of 7.5% compared to control mice that received a standard diet. Unpublished follow-on research on human neurons at the University of Central Florida is revealing that exposure to glutamate causes what appears to be wrinkling or entanglements of filaments which run in the axons. We will refer to this as varicosities. These varicosities block signal pathways between the muscle and the neuron. By adding AKG and GABA at 48 hours after exposure to the extracellular fluid, the varicosity is reversed.

---

17   The Deanna Protocol® added to a standard diet significantly extended survival time of SOD1-G93A mice by 7.5% (p = 0.001), Ari C, Poff AM, Held HE, Landon CS, Goldhagen CR, et al., "Metabolic Therapy with Deanna Protocol Supplementation Delays Disease Progression and Extends Survival in Amyotrophic Lateral Sclerosis (ALS) Mouse Model," *PLoS ONE*, 9(7) (2014); see http://dx.plos.org/10.1371/journal.pone.0103526.

Also, mitophagy has been seen under electron microscopy. Restoring mitochondria energy production restores mitochondrial morphology and membrane potential, and the functional capacity to generate ATP.[18] There is a mechanism, even if it is poorly understood at present, which reverses the damage to nerve cells when AKG and GABA is administered and reaches the motor neurons.

---

18 http://www.alzforum.org/news/research-news/als-parkinsons-proteins-co-mingle-mitochondria-destruction-pathway.

Chapter Fifteen

Science

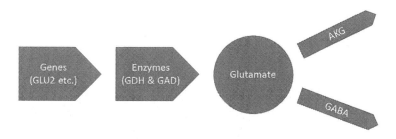

The authors' hypothesis is that, if the bodies of PALS can't metabolize glutamate, for whatever reason, then PALS lack whatever substances are produced by metabolizing glutamate. Why didn't anyone think of that before? While everyone else was looking at glutamate poisoning, and what could be done to get rid of excess glutamate, we decided to provide Deanna with nutritional supplementation of the substances missing from the failure of glutamate metabolizing in PALS, alpha-Ketoglutarate (AKG) and gamma-amino butyric acid (GABA).[19] These supplements

19   Berg J.M., Tymoczko J.L., Stryer L. (2002). Section 23.3.1. Alpha-Amino Groups Are Converted into Ammonium Ions by the Oxidative Deamination of Glutamate. *Biochemistry*, Stryer (Ed.), 5th Ed., W.H. Freeman and Company, New York; Baker P, et al. (1997). Determinants of Substrate Specificity in the Superfamily of Amino Acid Dehydrogenases. *Biochemistry* 36, 16109–16115; and Winnock, F., Ling, Z., De Proft, R., Dejonghe, S., Schuit, F., Gorus, F., & Pipeleers,

are widely available at comparatively low cost, and PALS have reported improvement by adding them to their diet.

Granted, this is a departure from orthodoxy. Granted, it was the authors' desperate attempt to have some impact, any impact, on this perplexing disease. To be clear, the authors agree that excess extracellular glutamate has the potential to poison surrounding cells in PALS. This has been studied by others in animal models and, at least in the spinal type of ALS, by human volunteers, comparing healthy volunteers and PALS.[20] According to Akiva Leibowitz et al., "excess of glutamate in the brain's extracellular fluids stimulates glutamate receptors, which in turn lead to cell swelling, apoptosis, and neuronal death."[21] This independent research does not contradict the results observed in PALS taking the Deanna Protocol®. To the contrary, the authors believe that toxic levels of extracellular glutamate cause spreading of ALS in PALS, but the Deanna Protocol® targets distressed neurons and helps to stop neuronal death and helps to reverse varicosities caused by excess glutamate.

D. (April 2002). Correlation between GABA release from rat islet β-cells and their metabolic state. *American Journal of Physiology— Endocrinology and Metabolism*, 282.4, 937–942.

20   Andreadou E., Kapaki E., Kokotis P., Paraskevas G.P., Katsaros N., Libitaki G., Petropoulou O., Zis V., Sfagos C., Vassilopoulos D. (2008). Plasma glutamate and glycine levels in patients with amyotrophic lateral sclerosis. *In Vivo*, 22, 137–141.

21   See Akiva Leibowitz, Matthew Boyko, Yoram Shapira, and Alexander Zlotnik. (2012). Blood Glutamate Scavenging: Insight into Neuroprotection. *Int J Mol Sci.*, 13.8) 10041–10066.

The authors have focused on ALS, but both human clinical studies and animal models have shown a pathological association between elevated glutamate in extracellular fluid, the fluid between neurons in the brain, and many neurodegenerative disorders, such as stroke[22], traumatic brain injury[23], intracerebral hemorrhage[24], brain hypoxia[25], glaucoma[26], HIV dementia[27], and malignant glioma[28]. The authors have received some testimonies from patients suffering from other neurological disorders, such as Alzheimer's, that the Deanna Protocol® helps them,

22   Castillo J., Davalos A., Naveiro J., Noya M. (1996). Neuroexcitatory amino acids and their relation to infarct size and neurological deficit in ischemic stroke. *Stroke*, 27:1060–1065.

23   Zauner A., Bullock R., Kuta A.J., Woodward J., Young H.F. (1996). Glutamate release and cerebral blood flow after severe human head injury. *Acta Neurochir. Suppl.*, 67:40–44.

24   Castillo J., Davalos A., Alvarez-Sabin J., Pumar J.M., Leira R., Silva Y., Montaner J., Kase C.S (2002). Molecular signatures of brain injury after intracerebral hemorrhage. *Neurology*, 58, 624–629.

25   Johnston M.V., Trescher W.H., Ishida A., Nakajima W. (2001). Neurobiology of hypoxic-ischemic injury in the developing brain. *Pediatr. Res.*, 49, 735–741.

26   Bunting H., Still R., Williams D.R., Gravenor M., Austin M.W. (2010). Evaluation of plasma glutamate levels in normal tension glaucoma. *Ophthalmic Res.*, 43:197–200.

27   Espey M.G., Basile A.S., Heaton R.K., Ellis R.J. (2002). Increased glutamate in CSF and plasma of patients with HIV dementia. *Neurology*, 58, 1439–1440.

28   Takano T., Lin J.H., Arcuino G., Gao Q., Yang J., Nedergaard M. (2001). Glutamate release promotes growth of malignant gliomas. *Nat. Med.*, 7, 1010–1015.

also. Winning the Fight, Inc. does not have the resources to test, adequately, the Deanna Protocol® in PALS, and has not been able to test the Deanna Protocol® in patients with these other neurodegenerative diseases. However, the testimonies of these other patients indicate that the Deanna Protocol® might act to interrupt the spreading of the damage caused by toxic levels of extracellular glutamate.

The National Institute of Health (NIH) funded a study for finding a substance to break down glutamate, and it was widely accepted that excess glutamate is associated with ALS.[29] Glutamate is elevated and GABA is diminished in the brain of human patients with ALS compared to healthy people.[30] Glutamate is an intermediate substance in the body that is naturally acted on by enzymes in healthy people. Glutamate dehydrogenase (GDH) and glutamate decarboxylase (GAD) are two of these enzymes. Unfortunately, synthetically compounding GDH in pill form would cost about $1,000 per gram. Worse still GDH is not stable. Additional work would need to be done to find a stable compound that could provide GDH and GAD to patients.

GDH and GAD enzymes are produced by the genes, such as GLUD2 and GAD1.[31] Now, there are many reasons

---

29   Redler R.L., & Dokholyan, N.V. (2012). The complex molecular biology of amyotrophic lateral sclerosis (ALS). *Prog Mol Biol Transl Sci.* 107, 215–62. http://www.ncbi.nlm.nih.gov/pubmed/22482452.

30   http://www.alzforum.org/news/research-news/brain-imaging-suggests-neurotransmitter-imbalance-als.

31   Plaitakis, A., Latsoudis, H., Kanavouras, K., Ritz, B., Bronstein,

that dysfunctional genes may not be producing sufficient quantities of these enzymes. Also, transcription errors may cause defective or inefficient enzymes to be produced in the body. Even if the enzymes are not produced defectively, something else in the body could act on these enzymes to cause them to fail to metabolize glutamate. Whatever the cause, excess extracellular glutamate is known to be associated with ALS. We now know the reason why glutamate is not being broken down. It's not because these enzymes are missing. It is because the glutamate is outside the cell where it may not be metabolized.

The authors do not discount the damage that excess glutamate can do, but there was nothing that could be done, in the short term, to restore Deanna's enzymatic break down of glutamate, and Deanna did not have time on her side. Instead of focusing on what could not be done, the authors decided to focus on what could be done, and replacing the substances that would be present if normal metabolic break down of glutamate occurred was a good place to start.

Before proceeding further, the authors find it necessary to warn against some of the therapies that they have found that don't work. While there is evidence that toxins play a role,[32] as an environmental factor, in ALS, chelation

J.M. et al. (Mar 2010). Gain-of-function Variant in GLUD2 Glutamate Dehydrogenase Modifies Parkinson's Disease Onset. *European Journal of Human Genetics*; 18.3, 336.

32   Woolsey P.B. (Nov 2008). Cysteine, sulfite, and glutamate toxicity: a cause of ALS? *J. Altern. Complement. Med.*, 14.9, 1159–64.

therapies have generally proven ineffective in staving off any of the symptoms of ALS or prolonging PALS lives. For that matter, until the discovery of the Deanna Protocol®, no therapy has been able to extend the lives of PALS more than a few months in clinical trials.

According to the NIH, in most cases, ALS "…is a multi-factorial disorder triggered by as yet unknown factors, including exposure to toxicants in the environment (either alone or in combination with specific genetic factors)."[33] These words are from the NIH, not the authors. Incidence and prevalence are observed to be generally uniform worldwide. NIH includes "mitochondrial dysfunction/oxidative stress" as one of four mechanisms responsible for cell death that is responsible for the symptoms of ALS. The other three are 1) altered/disrupted protein processing; 2) excitotoxicity/altered calcium homeostasis; and 3) altered cytoskeletal function/axonal transport. Mitochondrial dysfunction is the working hypothesis, but altered/disrupted protein processing is an equally valid hypothesis that would benefit from AAKG and GABA supplementation.

The authors believe that the studies sponsored by the Weizmann Institute and others sponsored by the NIH support a conclusion that ALS is a type of metabolic disorder and at some level, the metabolic disorder results in cell death and the release of glutamate into extracellular space, which spreads the disease throughout the central

---

33 https://grants.nih.gov/grants/guide/rfa-files/RFA-NS-04-003. html; The etiology, pathogenesis and treatment of ALS; August 8, 2003; RFA-NS-04-003.

nervous systems of PALS. The authors believe that the Deanna Protocol® provides energy to neurons in distress, by keeping them alive and interrupting the mechanism that causes spreading of ALS in PALS. Allowing neurons to survive when toxic levels of extracellular glutamate would otherwise cause irreversible neuronal cell death is a viable mechanism for the Deanna Protocol® in PALS. The authors argue that it is the cascade effect of toxic levels of extracellular glutamate that causes the spread of ALS in PALS. Anything that can interrupt the cascading spread of extracellular glutamate can benefit PALS. The substances provided in the Deanna Protocol® offer cells an alternative source of energy, allowing some of the cells to survive that would otherwise die, releasing their glutamate into the surrounding extracellular fluid. If enough cells survive, the level of glutamate in the extracellular fluid can be reduced by natural processes, slowing or stopping the progression of the disease.

Chapter Sixteen

Deanna's Testimony

The degeneration caused by ALS has stopped progressing rapidly as a direct result of the Deanna Protocol®. Some of the most frightening symptoms have reversed. I am regaining strength in my arms and legs. I don't become a rigid statue, anymore. I can carry a glass of water without spilling its contents. I can roll over in bed. I can talk well enough for people to understand me. I am able to fight back against ALS.

Let me explain how I know that it is the Deanna Protocol® that is making the difference. First, when I started taking AAKG and GABA, I was able to do what I could not do before. Second, when I ran out of AAKG, I lost the ability to do those things again, only to regain the ability when I started taking it again.

Third, I am sure that it is not a placebo, because I tried so many other remedies that failed to even slow the degeneration caused by ALS. Now, I can fight back and am stopping the loss of capabilities caused by ALS in its tracks. No, it is not a cure. Yes, it is keeping me in the game.

Fourth, I can exercise without exhausting my muscles by taking additional AKG before and during exercise. If I don't take enough AKG, muscle tremors and spasticity will result, but I can manage the amount that I am taking to prevent these symptoms.

Don't believe me. Try it yourself. If you are a neurologist, then let a patient try it. You'll see what a difference that it makes, if you don't wait until it is too late to help.

Chapter Seventeen

ALSFRS

If you don't believe the science and first person account, then at least believe the results of ALSFRS scores reported by PALS. Attached as Appendix A are graphs for PALS registered on www.winningthefight.org as users of the Deanna Protocol®. These PALS have voluntarily submitted ALSFRS scores via the website, and we thank them for doing this. We wish we had more, but both time and space are limited. The graphs can be interpreted by the following criteria:

- The "Onset of Symptom Date" is an ALSFRS Score of 48, and therefore the first score.
- Average decline for PALS not on the DP® is 1 point per month.
- Any decline less than 1 point per month is slower than average decline.
- PALS on the DP® were asked, periodically, to return to complete the ALSFRS.
- There was no way to ensure compliance with DP® recommendations.
- Less than half (only 6 of 34) scored 1 or greater; only 4 of 34 were greater than 1; 28 out of 34 were less than 1; and 14 of 34 were less than 0.5.

These self-reported ALSFRS scores are evidence of a delay in the progression of ALS in PALS attempting to comply with the recommendations of the Deanna Protocol®. On average, with a large enough statistical sample and a median equivalent to the mean, 17 PALS should have scores higher than one and 17 PALS should have scores lower than one. From the reported ALSFRS, many more PALS are lower than one than are greater than one. This indicates that these PALS are benefiting from whatever they are doing to implement the Deanna Protocol®. Realistically, compliance is not likely to be 100% with all of the recommendations given. So, the scores are an indication that some benefit is to be gained by reasonable attempts to comply. Only 4 of 34 are greater than the average rate of loss!

More resources are needed to collect ALSFRS scores from more PALS, preferably under the care of a neurologist, ensuring compliance and correct reporting of scores. While a clinical trial is neither ethical nor required, a study could be conducted to collect ALSFRS from neurology patients voluntarily complying with the Deanna Protocol®, with nothing more than a data collection plan and approval of an institutional review board. Winning the Fight, Inc. would welcome this type of study.

If you don't believe the ALSFRS scores reported by PALS, then at least believe the double blind study in SOD1-G93A mouse study conducted at the University of South

Florida.[34] Nothing works in these mice, except the Deanna Protocol®, and nothing currently available to PALS works as effectively as the Deanna Protocol®.

Winning the Fight, Inc. needs your help to reach PALS with this good news.

---

34 The Deanna Protocol® added to a standard diet significantly extended survival time of SOD1-G93A mice by 7.5% (p = 0.001), Ari C, Poff AM, Held HE, Landon CS, Goldhagen CR, et al., "Metabolic Therapy with Deanna Protocol Supplementation Delays Disease Progression and Extends Survival in Amyotrophic Lateral Sclerosis (ALS) Mouse Model," *PLoS ONE*, 9(7) (2014); see http://dx.plos.org/10.1371/journal.pone.0103526.

Chapter Eighteen

SOD1-G93A Mice

If you don't believe anything else, then at least believe the undeniable results of a blinded study in SOD1-G93A mice.

Dr. Mary Newport put Winning the Fight, Inc. in contact with Dr. Dominic D'Agostino at the University of South Florida (USF). Now, Dr. D'Agostino acts as liaison with USF's Neuroscience Department and has since become a key researcher supporting the benefits of the Deanna Protocol®. Winning the Fight, Inc. sponsored research in SOD1-G93A mice in Dr. D'Agostino's lab.

Dr. D'Agostino has significant research programs examining the effect of a ketogenic diet in treating other disorders, such as cancer. He was interested in how ketone bodies (KB's) impact other disorders, also, believing that a ketogenic diet might be an answer for other metabolic disorders, since KB's can enter the energy cycle in cells, as an alternative to the energy cycle that ordinarily produces 95% of the energy in the cells.[35]

Dr. D'Agostino is a brilliant scientist and innovative thinker with an inquisitive mind, not one to blindly accept the status quo. His attitude was a breath of fresh

---

35 Ernster, L; Dallner, G. (1995). Biochemical, physiological and medical aspects of ubiquinone function. *Biochimica et Biophysica Acta*, 1271.1, 195–204.

air, compared to some of the closed minds that the authors have encountered. This is not to say that Dr. D'Agostino did not have preconceived notions. He believed that the ketogenic diet was going to be successful in ALS mice. He chose the most difficult model, SOD1-G93A mice.

Since Deanna has already tried the ketogenic diet and it failed her, the authors were doubtful. Winning the Fight, Inc. compromised with Dr. D'Agostino, who developed a blinded research program designed to compare control mice to the core Deanna Protocol®, to a ketogenic diet and to a combination of the core Deanna Protocol® and a ketogenic diet. The core Deanna Protocol® tested on the mice was oral administration of AKG, GABA and Complex 1 (a combination of Ubiquinol and NADH).[36]

Orally administered caprylic acid was added to the experimental design to test oral administration of coconut oil. Caprylic acid did not improve the condition of SOD1-G93A mice.[37] Furthermore, the authors found a study done

---

36 Csilla Ari, Angela Poff, Heather Held, Tina Fiorelli, Craig Goldhagen and Dominic D'Agostino, "Increased TCA Cycle Intermediates In Response to Diet with Deanna Protocol in ALS Mouse Model," *The Journal of the Federation of American Societies for Experimental Biology* (FASEBJ) (2014); and See http://www.fasebj.org/content/28/1_Supplement/578.3?related-urls=yes&legid=fasebj;28/1_Supplement/578.3.

37 Success with the Deanna Protocol® in mice was first reported in 2013. Csilla Ari, Craig R. Goldhagen, Angela Poff, Heather Held, Carol Landon, Nicholas Mavromates, Dominic D. D'Agostino, "Effect of Alternative Metabolic Fuels as a Potential ALS Therapy in Mice and Humans," AHS Conference (2013). http://www.winningthefight.net/Content/Protocol/Atlanta_Poster_AHS_Conference_Draft_V1.pdf.

on ALS mice done by Wei Zhao and Pasinetti, which likewise concluded that orally administered caprylic acid did
not improve the outcome for the ALS mice.[38] A ketogenic
diet did not prolong the lives of ALS mice, and a ketogenic
diet or ketone bodies added to the core Deanna Protocol®
did not improve over the standard diet and Deanna Proto-
col®, either.[39]

Scientists theorize that the accumulation of mutant
SOD1 disrupts the functions of the cell by harming the
mitochondria and certain proteins. SOD1 mutations cause
only about 2% of human cases, causing critics to believe
that etiological mechanisms could be different from those
responsible for the sporadic side of ALS. For clinical studies, ALS-SOD1 mice continue to be the best model of
ALS but scientists continue to look to develop other more
useful models. One of the frustrations among scientists
is that nothing works to prolong the life spans of SOD1-
G93A mice, but then nothing worked in humans until the
Deanna Protocol®. Testing the DP in SOD1-G93A mice
seemed like a worthy challenge.

The SOD1 gene produces an enzyme called Cu/Zn
Superoxide Dismutase. The cause of ALS in humans

---

38 Zhao, W., Pasinetti, G.M. et al. (2012). Caprylic Triglycerides as a
Novel Therapeutic Approach to Effectively Improve the Performance
and Attenuate the Symptoms Due to the Motor Neuron Loss in ALS
Disease. *PLoS ONE* 7(11) (e49191).

39 Ari C, Poff AM, Held HE, Landon CS, Goldhagen CR, et al.,
"Metabolic Therapy with Deanna Protocol Supplementation Delays
Disease Progression and Extends Survival in Amyotrophic Lateral
Sclerosis (ALS) Mouse Model," *PLoS ONE*, 9(7) (2014).

remains unknown, but in 1993, scientists made a break-through that may prove important in finding a cure. The scientists discovered that mutations in the gene that pro-duces SOD1 were associated with 20% of the families that pass on a predisposition to ALS, genetically.

The enzyme SOD1 is an antioxidant that protects peo-ple from damage caused by super oxide which is a toxic, free radical formed in the mitochondria. These free radi-cals can damage the mitochondria as well as a cell's DNA and proteins within the cell. There can be cell death among several other possibilities. It is not known yet how motor neuron degeneration results from SOD1 gene mutation. But scientists believe that poor functioning of this gene may be due to an accumulation of free radicals. However, there is also research indicating that mutant SOD1 causes toxicity in another way.

Mice that lack the SOD1 gene usually do not get the disease, although they can show signs of muscle atrophy and shorter life spans. So the toxic properties of mutant SOD1-G93A could be due to a functional gain instead of a functional loss. Also, for both familial and sporadic ALS, a typical pathological result has been found to be an aggre-gation of proteins. For mutant SOD1 mice, aggregates of mutant SOD1 were discovered only in diseased tissues. When motor neurons degenerated, greater amounts were detected. This is perplexing. Why don't proteins accumu-late in healthy tissues? Does this invalidate the model or is this part of the disease?

Below is a graph of results from the initial study done on SOD1-G93A mice. The Deanna Protocol® (DP) was added to the standard diet (SD) that is fed to mice and to a special ketogenic diet (KD) that was fed to the mice. All of the mice lived to be 110 days old. The percentage of living mice on the standard diet (SD), alone, is represented by squares. These mice are considered controls, meaning they received no special treatment, and the control mice did the worst.

The SD+DP mice are represented by triangles and a broken line. These mice were fed the Deanna Protocol® and did the best of all of the mice both on testing and longevity. Many of the mice on the ketogenic diet (KD) died at nearly the same time as the control mice on a standard diet, but a few survived longer than their control counterparts, interestingly. Even more interestingly, the mice on both the ketogenic diet and the Deanna Protocol® (KD+DP),

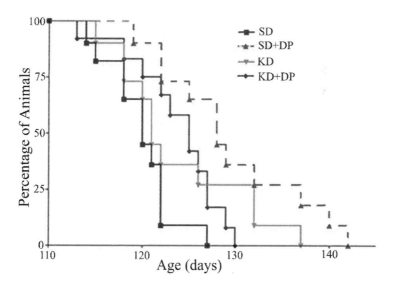

Figure A: Longevity of mice in the study sponsored by Winning the Fight, Inc.

represented by diamonds, died sooner than the mice on the standard diet and the Deanna Protocol® (SD+DP), represented by the broken line and triangles.

The results disclosed by the graph is striking but only covers longevity. What the complete results of the study show was that the ALS mice **did better on motor skills tests and lived longer on the Deanna Protocol®**, which is what Dr. Tedone has observed from Deanna and has heard from other PALS who have reported their ALSFRS scores on winningthefight.org. The authors are so thankful for those PALS who have voluntarily reported their scores on winningthefight.org, which have shown a remarkable slowing of the progression of their disease, when on the Deanna Protocol®. **We would like even more PALS to participate**. The more PALS who participate, the harder it is for mainstream neurologists to ignore these results.

Now, I know how hard it is to change a mindset that thinks that any type of dietary supplementation is merely quackery. But think a minute here. Nobody at Winning the Fight, Inc. has any incentive to make any of this up. Nobody at USF has any reason to make this up. In fact, USF's study showed that a ketogenic diet failed to improve mice scores or to prolong the lives of mice nearly as well as the Deanna Protocol®. Dr. D'Agostino's experimental design disproved his own hypothesis. So, bias did not figure into this study. Quite to the contrary. The study in ALS mice proved that the effects visible in human patients on the Deanna Protocol® were not merely isolated anecdotal evidence that can be conveniently dismissed.

No clinical trial is needed to place PALS on the Deanna Protocol®. All of the dietary supplements of the core Deanna Protocol® are readily available and not very expensive. All of the supplements are safe and are safely taken at the dosages recommended in the Deanna Protocol®. There is absolutely no reason not to recommend, clinically, the Deanna Protocol® to any patient that presents with symptoms of a neurological disease that might be ALS. There is every reason to encourage patients to phase in the Deanna Protocol® as early as possible, before irreversible damage is done by the cascade effect. No FDA approval is necessary for nutritional supplementation.

When the mouse studies described above were finished, Drs. Tedone and D'Agostino presented them at the Ancestral Health Symposium, the NEALS Conference, and the Society for Neuroscience conference. These results were presented again at the ALS Conference in Clearwater in October 2013. A summary of the conference in Clearwater failed to even mention our studies and our remarkable results with the Deanna Protocol®. In the same SOD1-G93A mouse model that our study used, many other treatments had been tested and *all* had failed to mitigate the effects of ALS. The Deanna Protocol® was the only treatment that succeeded. There were many questions and much interest after Dr. D'Agostino's presentation, but those in charge of reporting on the conference did not deem it important enough to mention in their summary.

Ultimately the research appeared as an open source

paper in July of 2014 so academia could critique the study.[40] Now, the paper and our outreach makes clear that **human patients** diagnosed with ALS have reported similar results to those observed in the double blind study of the SOD1-G93A mice. How did the mainstream ALS community respond? One clinician wrote:

> *I read the article and am glad to see these interesting approaches to therapy. I am always cautious about extrapolating the observations seen in the SOD1 mice to patients as we have seen numerous failures before over the last 20 years using this paradigm. Safety and efficacy, unfortunately, haven't translated well from animal models of ALS to humans but I am always hopeful.*

In the article and presentations, Dr. D'Agostino points out that *"What's unique about the Deanna Protocol® is that it hits multiple mechanisms working synergistically together to prevent the cells of the body from dying."* How did mainstream neurologists respond?

According to a September 2, 2014 story in USF's student newspaper, *The Oracle,* Dr. Lara Katzin, a neurologist at USF's own ALS Clinic, said that the clinic could not officially support the Deanna Protocol®. This is even more remarkable, because Dr. Katzin, herself, has examined

---

40   Ari C, Poff AM, Held HE, Landon CS, Goldhagen CR, et al., "Metabolic Therapy with Deanna Protocol Supplementation Delays Disease Progression and Extends Survival in Amyotrophic Lateral Sclerosis (ALS) Mouse Model," *PLoS ONE,* 9(7) (2014).

Deanna and returned a diagnosis of ALS. Dr. D'Agostino believes that the Deanna Protocol® is unique, because "...*it hits multiple mechanisms working synergistically together to prevent the cells of the body from dying.*" What does Dr. Katzin think? *The Oracle* quoted Dr. Katzin as saying that the Deanna Protocol® is "*...a whole list of different compounds being taken without individual ones being studied,*" and "*It's just not done in the way that regular clinical trials are done.*"[41] "*Patients can be vulnerable to anything put online that says it can make them better,*" Dr. Katzin said, according to *The Oracle.*

The blinded study in SOD1-G93A mice at USF is not putting anything online that could possibly deceive PALS. The study supports what PALS, themselves, have reported on winningthefight.org. Why is this even an issue for Dr. Katzin? The Deanna Protocol® benefits PALS. Why won't mainstream ALS researchers and neurologists accept evidence of this? The concept of "Group Think," alone, doesn't begin to explain the reaction.

Perhaps, cynicism begins to explain some of the reaction. A cynicism rooted in failure after failure over decades is so difficult to uproot. The authors did not have the luxury of cynicism. Deanna's life depended on willingness to stare failure straight in the face, and to keep on trying. Love conquers cynicism. At least it did in Deanna and her dad, a team who have never known how to quit, even with odds stacked high against success. Sure, the authors

---

41 http://www.usforacle.com/news/view.php/845337/USF-researchers-take-on-true-ALS-challen.

made mistakes, trying to understand the disease ravaging Deanna's body. Deanna tried things that didn't work, and the chelation treatments might have done more harm than good. But stubborn perseverance and determination to find something that could slow the progression of Deanna's disease won out. Everything that could be learned about ALS was needed to find a treatment, and the authors continue to learn, to look and to work on a way of reversing the damage that ALS has done to Deanna. Cynicism has no room in a father's heart.

In the case of Dr. Katzin, not even cynicism can explain her stubborn refusal to believe the evidence produced by researchers at her own university. You can see from her response that no study, other than a clinical study of human patients designed for testing a single drug, could even hope to persuade her. However, the authors and Dr. D'Agostino both believe that it is the synergistic effect of a combination of nutritional supplements in the Deanna Protocol® that provides the surprising benefits to PALS. Any single substance, isolated from the others, would not be as effective.

Also, how could any researcher ethically enroll PALS into a double blind clinical trial that would give some of them mere placebos, when the authors already know that the Deanna Protocol® works and is safe? The nutritional supplements are not drugs. Anybody can buy them, now. They are readily available and safe. As common supplements, the substances recommended in the Deanna Protocol® are not very expensive. How could anyone ethically deny PALS the nutrition that their bodies need to function better?

Chapter Nineteen

Dr. D'Agostino's Testimony

I was traveling in Europe for about two weeks; when I came back there were messages on my answering machine. A bunch of them, actually. Dr. Tedone's was by far the most heart-wrenching, describing his daughter Deanna as having ALS and his investigation of different diets and different metabolic therapies for the treatment of her disease. He came across me through a mutual friend, Dr. Mary Newport. He also knew that I was developing and testing ketone bodies for neurological disorders and cancer. His message told me about the results that he observed in Deanna with the use of metabolic therapy that he called the Deanna Protocol®. I was intrigued, but reasonably skeptical.

I spoke with Dr. Tedone about the science behind the Deanna Protocol® by phone. Then, I went over to his house. I met Deanna and her family. I wanted to do everything that I could within my capability and to connect them with other people who had expertise in this area. The science made sense to me. I had experience with metabolomics, ketones and ketone bodies. What Dr. Tedone was describing was not new to me, except for the connection with ALS.

I am a scientist. I like to test a good, testable hypothesis. The sequence was unusual. Winning the Fight had success in human ALS patients, already. Now, I was asked to test the hypothesis in the lab. Usually, it is the other way around. Metabolic therapy refers to use of the body's own metabolism, i.e., the substances naturally found in the body to supply it energy and to regenerate or replenish the body's cells. This therapy gives the body what it cannot, for whatever reason, supply for itself or we take advantage of the body's natural processes to treat it. The field is termed Metabolomics.

Through trial and error and some research, Deanna and Dr. Tedone determined that ALS could be treated with ketones. There were several determining factors in finding something that would work to help Deanna manage her disease: Deanna had a father that could make sense out of sometimes conflicting and contradictory literature published about ALS, the substances that were chosen are considered non-harmful and naturally occurring, and there was no other treatment available for ALS that held any promise for a better outcome.

Now, I teach biochemistry to medical students. Ordinarily, there is no significant depth of exposure to nutritional biochemistry and metabolomics in a general medical school curriculum. So, it is not surprising that doctors don't understand metabolomics, unless they choose to specialize in this area. I don't think that neurologists are ready to accept that a patient with ALS can manage this disease by diet. So, there is going to be a natural resistance to any claims that metabolomics delays the progression of ALS.

However, the response that Dr. Tedone described

to me fit what I understand from a metabolic physiology perspective. I wanted to know more. We engaged in many discussions by phone and email. I participate in conference calls with the board of Winning the Fight, Inc. every couple of weeks, when I can. I could understand his frustration with clinical doctors, and I had to respect his perseverance, when he and his family were alone in thinking that they could have an impact on this disease.

The Deanna Protocol® is a comprehensive therapy that involves nutritional supplements, physiotherapy, coconut oil massage and intravenous glutathione. The glutathione is an antioxidant intended to reduce oxidative stress in PALS. The physiotherapy is to increase muscle strength and mass in order to reverse some of the muscle atrophy caused by ALS. The coconut oil massage has been helpful in increasing muscle mass in some PALS. However, the core components of the Deanna Protocol® are the supplements taken orally, AAKG, GABA, Ubiquinol, niacin and 5-hydroxytryptophan.

What I tested was the core supplements that could be administered orally to the mice. Obviously, we can't do a coconut oil massage, physiotherapy or intravenous glutathione in a double blind study in mice. We added arginine – alpha ketoglutarate, GABA, soluble CoQ10 and caprylic acid in a standard diet that already included niacin. I was interested in the ketogenic diet, also. I have used this diet to treat other diseases, and I thought it might work as an alternative source of energy for motor neurons in PALS.

This mouse model exhibits loss of motor function in the hind limbs that is similar to human patients with ALS. Usually, one limb weakens first, then two limbs and visible tremors. There's a set of criteria that researchers follow to characterize the progression of the disease in the mice. Researchers observe the mice daily and record their findings based on markings unique to each mouse, without knowing which mice are receiving the Deanna Protocol® and which aren't. The mice are tested for motor skills.

Using this double-blinded study method, the study found statistically significant delays in the progression of the pathology of the SOD1-G93A mice eating the standard diet supplemented by the Deanna Protocol®. There is no doubt that it extended the survival of the mice. As far as I know, nothing else has worked with SOD1-G93A mice. I was surprised by the results, even though I knew that human PALS are benefiting.

Each day, the mice were given motor function tests such as a grip test, a hanging wire test and a rotarod test, which is a performance test based on a rotating rod with forced motor activity being applied. This study was very tedious and quite labor-intensive. Multiple trials of each mouse were required as strength; endurance and capacity to run were all tested. Multiple people did tests on each mouse in a blind study to assure accuracy of the test scores.

If you refer to the key to the right of the graph, you will see four acronyms. **SD** stands for mice that were on a standard diet and not being treated for ALS. **SD+DP** stands for mice that were on a standard diet and the Deanna

Protocol®. **KD** stands for mice that were on the ketogenic diet. **KD+DP** stands for mice that were on the ketogenic diet and the Deanna Protocol® simultaneously. The graph of Figure B shows strength and motor performance, measured by the ability of mice to hang on a wire for a certain amount of time. Figure A depicts survival rate, as previously shown.

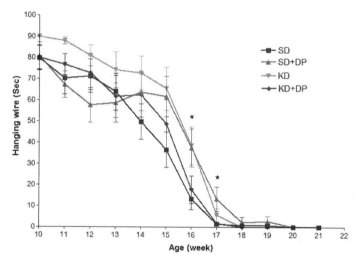

Figure B

The idea in our study was to test the ketogenic diet and also test it against the Deanna Protocol®. We fed the mice a standard diet, a standard diet supplemented by the Deanna Protocol®, a ketogenic diet and a combination of the ketogenic diet supplemented by the Deanna Protocol®. The standard diet supplemented by the Deanna Protocol® gave the best results. That was surprising to me. I expected more from the ketogenic diet or the combination of ketogenic and Deanna Protocol®.

My original hypothesis was that there would be some kind of additive effect by adding the ketogenic diet to the Deanna Protocol®. I expected the ketogenic diet to confer a neuro-protective effect by elevating blood ketone levels. This effect was published by others. We didn't see that. In ALS animal models, calorie restriction can accelerate the pathology in the mice. I'm not sure if the mice on the ketogenic diet received as may calories as those on the standard diet supplemented by the Deanna Protocol®. Other researchers discount this hypothesis, believing that mice will eat anything if they are hungry enough. I would like to know why the ketogenic diet didn't provide an additive benefit, as I expected, but the extent of the benefits from adding the Deanna Protocol® to the standard diet are quite surprising.

We presented preliminary findings at *The Ancestral Health Conference in Atlanta* and elsewhere. The preliminary results generated interest and a good deal of discussion. We incorporated some of the suggestions from the audience into the study. No other treatment has ever extended the life of SOD1-G93A mice, before. So, those familiar with the model were very interested in seeing a comparison between the metabolomics of the motor neuron cells of the DP mice and the standard diet mice. So, we sent out samples for testing. The results were very interesting.

For example, electron microscopy revealed the cells of the mice on the standard diet and Deanna Protocol® had mitochondria present in the nucleus. The cells from the mice on the standard diet alone, ketogenic diet alone and ketogenic diet plus the DP had no mitochondria present in the nucleus. Somehow the DP preserved the mitochondria in the nucleus, when the other diets did not.

Metabolic analysis by a third party lab revealed that the mice treated by the Deanna Protocol® had an increase of high energy phosphate bonds in motor neurons, compared to cells in other mice. We suppose that the AKG supplementation caused this. What we know is the DP mice had a substantial build-up of the energy cycle in motor neurons compared to other mice.

Metabolic analysis showed that phosphatidylcholine (PC) appeared to be remodeled for incorporation into cellular membranes and/or broken down into the free fatty acids glycerol and choline. Phosphatidylcholine was also seen to be in excess in the mice on the Deanna Protocol®. Although this was not a component of the core Deanna Protocol®. The increase in phosphatidylcholine seen in the Deanna Protocol® mice could be from ruptured membranes of dead cells.

Elevated levels of intermediates of fatty acid oxidation (FAO) and ready FAO substrates in the DP mice indicates increased beta-oxidation in response to supplementation of the standard diet with the Deanna Protocol®.

GABA and arginine in the Deanna Protocol® mice were at increased levels, and the levels of derivatives of GABA and arginine were elevated *in vivo*, also. We saw a decrease in spasticity of the DP mice, probably as a result of the GABA supplementation. This parallels observations from Deanna, suggesting that the SOD1-G93A model is an appropriate model for testing outcomes in humans.

We added arginine as a fellow traveler in the Deanna Protocol®. It is a basic amino acid and was needed to neutralize the acidic AKG. We also know that arginine increases the blood supply by causing vasodilation (widens arteries). The metabolic study indicated there is an increase in arginine in the serum of the mice treated with the Deanna Protocol®. The effect of arginine on vasodilation is known. So, we suppose that this might have facilitated removal of excess glutamate from Deanna Protocol® treated mice.

An increased presence of fatty acid metabolites evidences increased metabolism in the mice cohort treated with the Deanna Protocol® as opposed to other cohorts. Apparently, the DP mice had increased cellular energy production in the mitochondria of motor neurons, providing a supercharged metabolism compared to motor neurons of other cohorts.

All of this supports the original hypothesis of Dr. Tedone. None of it disproves it. The research raises questions about why a ketogenic diet doesn't help more, but these questions are not central to the efficacy or safety of the Deanna Protocol®. Any clinical neurologist counseling patients with symptoms of a neurodegenerative disease needs to recommend the Deanna Protocol®, and assist patients with compliance.

PART THREE

The Deanna Protocol®

Chapter Twenty

The Deanna Protocol®
Program for ALS

This program and the Deanna Protocol® have been evolving as we receive input from our PALS base and research on ALS mice.

<u>**PLEASE READ ENTIRE DOCUMENT TO UNDERSTAND THE PROGRAM.**</u>

I. <u>**The Deanna Protocol® (DP)**</u>: The benefit of the substances in the DP has been documented by anecdotal evidence and our research on transgenic mice. The DP consists of 3 components: AKG, Complex 1 (consisting of Ubiquinol and NADH), and GABA.

<u>SUPPLEMENT</u>	<u>DOSAGE</u>	<u>PURPOSE</u>
AAKG	Begin with standard dosage on bottle and increase slowly to 18g/day.	Delivers energy to nerves

AKG	300 mg pills take approx. every hour (you are awake) between doses of AAKG. May be listed as alpha keto-glutaric acid	Delivers energy to nerves
Tryptophan	50 mg 1x/day (take at PM with niacin)	5-hyroxytryptophan is a precursor to NADH and also serotonin and melatonin, both inhibitory neuro-transmitters
Niacin (Non Flush)	250 mg 1x/day	Precursor to NADH
GABA	250 mg 2x/day	Inhibitory neurotransmitter
Ubiquinol*	400 mg 3x/day	CoQ10 helps energy cycle in mitochondria
*Optional		

A. <u>**Alpha Ketoglutarate [AKG] and Arginine Alpha Ketoglutarate [AAKG]**</u>: AKG is a key supplement to providing energy to the cells.

- We suggest both AAKG and AKG for the following reasons: 1) **<u>AAKG,</u>** due to the arginine, is more palatable and easier on the stomach. The arginine allows you to receive a larger dose of the AKG with minimal stomach discomfort. However, arginine has limitations; if you exceed 18g of arginine AKG per day, it may cause stomach and intestinal discomfort. The arginine also produces nitrous oxide (NO), a free radical. This may have unwanted side effects. A side effect of NO is swelling of the lower extremities, which is already a side effect in ALS. Arginine can also aggravate a preexisting heart condition. Arginine can also activate the Herpes simplex virus. Arginine also may have beneficial effects in ALS. Recent research reveals that when cells die they release glutamate into the extracellular space (space between cells). This glutamate causes the death of nearby cells. Blood vessel cells in contact with nerve tissue absorb the glutamate and pass it into the circulating blood. Since the NO produced by arginine increases blood flow by dilating blood vessels NO might be beneficial by helping to remove glutamate from the nerve tissue by increasing blood flow to the area. Future research will attempt to determine the value of arginine. 2) **Plain AKG** does not have arginine and will allow you to continuously deliver energy to nerve and muscle cells in between doses of AAKG. AKG is less palatable and harder on the stomach, but manageable in smaller doses.

- NOTE: AKG is an important source of energy for nerve and muscle cells. We do not know how long the AAKG or AKG remain in the body. Our goal is to make sure the body has AAKG or AKG in it whenever the cells need energy.

- AKG/AAKG DOSE—The dose is determined by the amount needed to suppress muscle symptoms [fasciculations, twitching, and cramps]. Based on reports from PALS and laboratory research, on average, a minimum of 16–18g of AAKG is required to have an effect. AAKG may cause diarrhea and bloating. Our experience has found that if you start with a low dose and gradually increase the dose not to exceed 18 grams over time these symptoms may be lessened or will stop. **Do not** take total dose at one time. Deanna takes 18g of AAKG and divides it between breakfast, lunch and dinner. In addition, she takes 4,300mg capsules of AKG every 1hr–1.5hrs between doses of AAKG up until bedtime. For the reasons stated above, if you need to increase the dose of AKG to decrease muscle symptoms, use AKG not AAKG. If you are very active, you may notice an increase in muscle symptoms. This means you have used up your energy supply and likely need more AKG.

- AKG is a supplement your body requires daily to keep cells alive. Your body does not store it or build a reserve. So taking it daily is essential. Please note with AAKG and AKG you may not notice an immediate change but changes should occur over time and may be subtle such as lessening of spasms, twitches/fasciculations, saliva, etc.

B. The AAKG you buy should have a 1:1 ratio of arginine to alpha keto-glutarate (manufactured by Prima Force® or Simplesa®). Most people tolerate it, but some people can't tolerate it. If you find the AAKG with the 1:1 ratio causes gastritis even after giving your body time to adjust then use the AAKG with a 2:1 ratio.

C. **Complex 1:** Complex 1 consists of the substances needed in the metabolism of AKG in the Krebs cycle (energy cycle).

   a. Ubiquinol is a more potent form of CoQ10. The most effective form Idebenone has been taken off the market. Thus, it is unavailable, except by prescription and very expensive. Laboratory data suggests taking 1,000mg–1,400mg of Ubiquinol daily. If a more effective form, such as, Idebenone is used less may be required.

   b. NADH is not able to be absorbed by the GI system, which is why the DP consists of niacin, a precursor to NADH, which can be absorbed by the GI system. Another precursor to NADH is 5-hydroxytryptophane [5-HTP].

D. **Gamma Amino Butyric Acid (GABA):** GABA is the primary inhibitory neuro transmitter and is recommended to counteract the spasticity and rigidity caused by the quantity of GABA being diminished. Grogginess is a possible side effect.

- Dose-changes according to the degree of spasticity present in the individual with ALS. Deanna takes 250 mg 2 times per day. If she feels more spastic, has tremors, cramps, or rigidity she increases the dose.

NOTE: Before you begin the protocol, take note of all your symptoms especially your muscle symptoms i.e. muscle twitching, tremors, spasms, etc. If after taking the Deanna Protocol® for 1 to 3 months, and you doubt that the protocol is beneficial, stop it for a few days and notice the difference in your muscle symptoms. If the symptoms worsen or increase, you know the protocol is working. Beginning the protocol again, should diminish the symptoms.

Please note we have included the following as part of the Deanna Protocol® Program for ALS. They are NOT part of the Deanna Protocol®.

II. **Antioxidants: Glutathione (GSH):** GSH is the most effective nervous system antioxidant known to man. The best delivery system for GSH is an IV 3000 mg once a week. The dose is determined by what is currently used by neurologists and wellness clinics. GSH can be delivered by suppository, Liposomal GSH, and sustained release GSH (sold by Thorne Research). Deanna gets the IV and takes sustained release GSH. In recommending this, we have accepted a large amount of research indicating the effectiveness of GSH in neutralizing ROS (reactive oxygen species) which we know are detrimental to nerve cells.

III. **Exercise:** Suggested respiratory therapy, speech therapy, personal training and/or physical therapy (not to exhaustion)—including active range of motion exercises, progressive resistance exercises (PRE), strengthening exercises, aerobic exercises, hand exercises, stretching to maintain joint mobility. PALS on the Deanna Protocol® have reported improvement with PRE. Therefore, we suggest doing strengthening exercises, but not to exhaustion (the point at which you can't use the muscle).

IV. **Massage:** Massage with extra virgin coconut oil. Anecdotal evidence reveals that muscle strength and size can be improved with this regimen. We have anecdotal evidence that massage with coconut oil can increase the size of atrophic muscles. Once per day, massage oil into muscles that have atrophied or diminished. Massage oil over entire body twice a week. The coconut oil is absorbed through the skin and supplies energy directly to the cells in muscles and nerves.

V.   **Oxaloacetate:** Research has shown that oxaloacetate is a supplement that neutralizes extra cellular glutamate, which is responsible for nerve cell death. Unfortunately, it only stays in the body for 15 to 30 minutes. It would be ideal to take one capsule every hour. The only manufacturer we found that makes it is Natural Dynamix and the product name is Endure DX.

Ancillary Supplements

These are **NOT** part of the Deanna Protocol® Program for ALS because we have not done research on these substances and don't have anecdotal evidence of their benefit. However, since they are recommended by the NIH we felt we should mention them.

These supplements can be supplied by a healthy diet, but PALS may need more than the normal population. The proper dose for ALS patients is unknown. The

NIH has published a manuscript "Nutrition and Supplements in Motor Neuron Diseases." Please refer to this document for details http://www.ncbi.nlm.nih.gov/pmc/articles/PMC2631353/. These supplements come in various forms. For example, Deanna takes B12 orally and via IV or injection.

*Please note not all companies make quality supplements. It is important to get good quality supplements. Your local health food store or wellness clinic should be able to advise you regarding good quality supplements. Some of the people taking the supplements have purchased from the following companies: Thorne Research, Life Extension, Prima Force®, Simplesa®, Kirkman Labs, Natural Dynamix and NOW. WINNING THE FIGHT, INC. does not endorse these companies, and there are likely other companies that sell quality supplements.

Chapter Twenty-One

Overview & Disclaimer

The supplement list, protocol questionnaire and any other information provided is not intended to treat, cure or prevent any condition or disease. The combination of supplements provided has not been tested in clinical trials, is not registered with the FDA and is not marketed as a drug. Please consult with your own physician or health care practitioner regarding the supplements and supplement list, questionnaire and any other information provided. You should always speak with a practitioner before taking any dietary, nutritional, herbal or homeopathic supplement. Supplements and other products are manufactured and distributed by third parties, and WINNING THE FIGHT, INC., does not independently test supplements and other products or confirm information provided by any third party, including, but limited, distributors and manufacturers. WINNING THE FIGHT, INC., shall have no liability to you, including, without limitation, any liability for any defective products. WINNING THE FIGHT, INC. makes no warranty, express or implied, with respect to any products or services, including any warranty of merchantability or fitness for a particular purpose. Under no circumstances, including, but not limited to negligence, shall WINNING THE FIGHT, INC. be liable for any direct, indirect, special, incidental or consequential damages, arising out of the use, or the inability to use, the supplements, supplement list, questionnaire and any other information provided. We do not warranty and shall have no liability regarding information provided regarding recommendations for supplements for any and all health purposes. This information is provided solely as information to use when discussing a regimen with your healthcare practitioners. WINNING THE FIGHT, INC. is providing this supplement list, questionnaire and any other information on an "as is" basis and makes no representations or warranties of any kind with respect to this or its contents. WINNING THE FIGHT, INC., nor any of its directors, officers, employees, contributing physicians, medical liaison, researchers, volunteers or other representatives will be held liable for damages arising out of or in connection with the use of the supplements, supplement list, questionnaire and any other information provided. This is a comprehensive limitation of liability that applies to all damages of any kind, including (without limitation) compensatory, direct, indirect or consequential damages, loss of data, income or profit, loss of or damage to property, bodily injury, and claims of third parties. It is imperative that you speak with practitioner before buying or using supplements. Each person is different, and the way someone reacts to a particular product may be significantly different from another. You should always speak with a practitioner before taking any dietary, nutritional, herbal or homeopathic supplement.

Chapter Twenty-Two

AKG

AKG is formed by one of two enzymatic reactions in the body, oxidative decarboxylation of isocitrate or oxidative deamination of glutamate. The chemical structure of the alpha-ketoglutaric acid is shown below:

AKG is essential to the energy cycle that takes place within the mitochondria of cells. It is a link in the cycle that provides energy to the cells.

Providing supplementation of those nutritional substances lacking from the failure of glutamate breaking down did not come to the authors as a flash of genius in the middle of the night. The authors were looking at glutamate poisoning too. The Deanna Protocol® came about through desperation. Nothing was working to help Deanna. There was nothing that the authors could contribute to gene therapy or enzymatic therapy. If you are to learn anything about Dr. Vince Tedone and Deanna Tedone-Gage, however, you must know that giving up never crosses their mind. Study. Try. Learn. Apply what you learn, and start all over again.

AKG is a ketone. A ketone is any organic compound with the structure: $\underset{R}{\overset{O}{\|}}_{R'}$ where the R and R' are carbon or carbon-containing groups. Below, the ketone in AKG is outlined in a dashed line, where the unlabeled vertices are all carbon atoms:

AKG is an important link in every cell's energy cycle (also called the citric acid cycle, Krebs cycle or tricarboxylic acid cycle). This energy cycle is a complex branched chain of bio-chemical reactions occurring within each cell and depends on enzymes and cofactors within organelles called the mitochondria. If the energy cycle in a cell becomes dysfunctional, the cell will die.

The circle in the drawing below represents a cell. This simple representation of an eukaryotic cell is shown with a single organelle. The oval-shaped boundary represents a lipid bilayer separating the interior of the organelle from the rest of the cell. As shown by the Acetyl-CoA shown entering the organelle, the lipid bilayer may allow transfer of substances from the organelle and into the organelle. Typical eukaryotic cells, including the cells of humans, may have many organelles. Among the organelles in

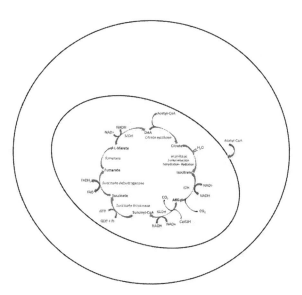

human cells are the mitochondria, sometimes referred to as the power houses of the cells. In the drawing, the oval organelle represents one of the mitochondria in a cell. Some cells contain several mitochondria. The mitochondria have their own DNA, separate and apart from the nuclear DNA of a human cell.

The mitochondria organelles are complex machines that produce most of the energy for the cells. If the energy cycle in the mitochondria breaks down, the cells are starved for energy. Based on research, the authors hypothesized that Deanna's body lacked enough AKG due to an interruption in the metabolism of glutamate. Could this hypothesis be disproven? Fortunately, a version of arginine-AKG (AAKG) was readily available as a dietary supplement, often used by body builders. Deanna started taking it. Her story is detailed in the earlier chapters of this book. Taking AKG had a dramatic effect on Deanna's quality of life. Deanna is able to do, now, what she had not been able to do for some time.

Tellingly, when Deanna's supply of AKG ran out, her symptoms returned. When Deanna recommenced the Deanna Protocol®, she felt better, again. The authors know that this is just anecdotal evidence, but it is compelling anecdotal evidence. The hypothesis was not disproven! In fact, Deanna's story is compelling evidence that arginine-AKG (AAKG) supplementation should be started as soon as possible for any patient who might have ALS. Her story has been repeated, again and again, by PALS reporting their own results with the Deanna Protocol® on www.winningthefight.org.

Finally, something worked, when nothing was working. The mechanism for how the Deanna Protocol® works can be explained in detail. It makes sense. There is a clear, understandable mechanism for how AKG supplementation works to provide the cells the energy that they need. And there is additional evidence. Deanna knows that when she exercises, she has to take more AKG in order to avoid muscle symptoms. Her cells, at least those cells in distress, need the extra AKG that is not being produced due to dysfunctional metabolism of glutamate or dysfunctional protein synthesis of some type.

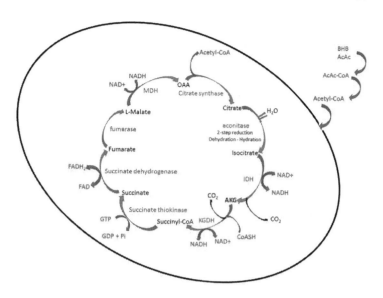

The organelle represented above schematically shows the energy cycle that occurs in the mitochondria in human eukaryotic cells. Production of AKG is an important step in the energy cycle. In the drawing, AKG is shown in the lower right quadrant of the cycle, between isocitrate and succinyl-CoA. Isocitrate dehydrogenase acts on isocitrate to produce AKG within the energy cycle. An alternative pathway for production of AKG is to enzymatically metabolize glutamate. PALS have excessive levels of extracellular glutamate, indicating that something interferes with the metabolic process needed to de-aminate glutamate, which is essential for this alternative pathway of AKG production.

Metabolic treatment for ALS is not a widely accepted treatment. Dr. Richard Veech, a world premier micro-biochemist at NIH, wrote a paper in 1980 in which he revealed that ketone bodies could stop nerve cells from degeneration.[42] Dr. Tedone asked Dr. Veech why nobody has tried AKG. He responded, *"Because the polarity of AKG will not allow it to cross the cell membrane into the cell, whereas the polarity of the ketone bodies [B-H-B, AcAc] allows them to cross the cell membrane."*[43] Dr. Tedone asked him, *"Suppose that the cell was dying. Would the polarity of the membrane change, therefore allowing the AKG to cross it?"* Dr. Veech replied, simply, *"yes."* Why didn't anyone ask this question before? This is a possible reason that AKG is more effective than ketone bodies in studies sponsored by Winning the Fight, Inc. AKG goes directly to cells in distress, while ketone bodies are spread thin by being able to cross all cell membranes. Now, the authors have proved effectiveness of AKG in SOD1-G93A mice, but our proof is falling on deaf ears, as of yet.

Winning the Fight, Inc. knows that many clinicians and researchers will be skeptical. Deanna is a single person. This is anecdotal evidence. You've heard this all before. Many PALS and patients with other neurodegenerative

---

42 Cahill, Jr., G.F., Beech, R.L., (2003). Ketoacids? Good medicine?" *Transactions of the American Clinical and Climatological Association*, 114, 149–163. http://www.ncbi.nlm.nih.gov/pmc/articles/PMC2194504/pdf/tacca00002-0213.pdf.

43 MacKenzie, E., Selak, M.A., Tennant, D.A., Payne, L.J., Crosby, S., Frederiksen, C.M., Watson, D.G., & Gottlieb, E. (2007). Cell-permeating Alpha-ketoglutarate Derivatives Alleviate Pseudohypoxia In Succinate Dehydrogenase-deficient Cells. *Molecular Cellular Biology*, 27.9, 3282–3289. http://mcb.asm.org/content/27/9/3282.

diseases have now adopted the Deanna Protocol® and have reported similar results when taking AKG.[44] Deanna did not benefit from the other diets and supposed remedies that she attempted, such as the KD, before she started taking the Deanna Protocol®. The KD and other suggestions proved ineffective. Only the Deanna Protocol® worked for Deanna and thousands of PALS, worldwide, who have now tried the Deanna Protocol®.

The authors have no reason to lie. Nobody at Winning the Fight, Inc. is receiving any salary or payment of any kind. This is a labor of love. The love of a father for his daughter and the love of the Tedone family for all the PALS suffering from ALS. They have seen its devastating effects first hand. Word needs to get out, so that other fathers and other daughters can experience the same hope that the Deanna Protocol® has brought to Deanna and her family and thousands of other PALS who found www.winningthefight.org.

The Deanna Protocol® started with Deanna taking AKG and other supplements. The Deanna Protocol® rapidly evolved, based on clinical feedback from Deanna, other PALS and patients with other neurodegenerative diseases. We have received feedback from physicians, thank you. And Winning the Fight, Inc. has sponsored research at the University of South Florida (USF). We appreciate all

---

44 A non-scientific survey was conducted by Winning the Fight, Inc. in November 2014, and 50 of 59 people who voluntarily responded reported some positive results from adding the Deanna Protocol® recommendations to their diet.

of the PALS who post on Winning the Fight's forum (www. winningthefight.org). We have learned a great deal from you about what works and what doesn't work. Many PALS are very knowledgeable and are adept at fine-tuning the Deanna Protocol® to their specific needs. Keep sending us your feedback.

Researchers at USF believed that the ketogenic diet (KD) would benefit ALS patients. Winning the Fight, Inc. provided research comparing the KD and the Deanna Protocol® to controls, mice on an ordinary diet. To the surprise of the researchers, the mice on KD, with or without supplementation by the Deanna Protocol®, showed less improvement in longevity than those on the standard diet with supplementation by the Deanna Protocol®.[45] The SOD1-G93A mice on the Deanna Protocol® did show improvement during testing of motor skills and for longevity compared to control mice and mice on the KD. The research was carefully done to avoid bias. If researchers had any preconceived bias, it would have favored mice on the KD. Nonetheless, the research confirmed the effects of the Deanna Protocol® already observed in human PALS.

CAUTION: Start out gradually, adding additional AAKG three times per day until you are taking enough

---

45 The Deanna Protocol® added to a standard diet significantly extended survival time of SOD1-G93A mice by 7.5% (p = 0.001), Ari C, Poff AM, Held HE, Landon CS, Goldhagen CR, et al., "Metabolic Therapy with Deanna Protocol Supplementation Delays Disease Progression and Extends Survival in Amyotrophic Lateral Sclerosis (ALS) Mouse Model," PLoS ONE, 9(7) (2014); see http://dx.plos.org/10.1371/journal.pone.0103526.

AAKG to prevent fasciculations and twitching, when at rest. AKG can cause stomach upset and diarrhea. Don't take more than 18 grams of AAKG per day, unless prescribed by a doctor. There are other sources of AKG that do not include arginine, and these can be taken before and during exercise, if additional AKG is needed. Care must be taken if swallowing is difficult to avoid choking hazard.

The AAKG you buy should have a 1:1 ratio of arginine to alpha Keto-glutarate (to our knowledge, Prima Force® and Simplesa® are the only two companies that manufacture AAKG with a 1:1 ratio). Most people tolerate it, but some people can't tolerate it. If you find the AAKG with the 1:1 ratio causes gastritis even after giving your body time to adjust then use the AAKG with a 2:1 ratio.

PALS, who have a cardiac condition should consult with their cardiologist or treating physician before taking AAKG as the nitrous oxide in arginine increases stress on the heart.

We suggest both AAKG and AKG for the following reasons: 1) **AAKG**, due to the arginine, is more palatable and easier on the stomach. The arginine allows you to receive a larger dose of the AKG with minimal stomach discomfort. However, arginine has limitations; if you exceed 18g of arginine AKG per day, it may cause stomach and intestinal discomfort. The arginine also produces nitrous oxide (NO) a free radical and may produce unwanted side effects. A side effect of NO is swelling of the lower extremities, which is already a side effect in ALS. Arginine can also aggravate a preexisting heart condition. Arginine can also activate the Herpes Simplex Virus. Arginine also may have beneficial effects in ALS. Recent research reveals that when cells die they release glutamate into the extracellular space (space between cells). This glutamate causes the death of nearby cells. Blood vessel cells in contact with nervous tissue absorb the glutamate and pass it into the circulating blood. Since the NO produced by arginine increases blood flow by dilating blood vessels NO might be beneficial by helping to remove glutamate from the nerve tissue by increasing blood flow to the area. Future research will attempt to determine the value of arginine. 2) **Plain AKG** does not have arginine and will allow you to continuously deliver energy to nerve and muscle cells in between doses of AAKG. AKG is less palatable and harder on the stomach, but manageable in smaller doses.

IMPORTANT: THE AMOUNT OF AKG NEEDED BY PALS DEPENDS ON THE PATIENT AND THE LEVEL OF ACTIVITY OF THE PATIENT. ADJUST AS NEEDED.

AKG/AAKG DOSE—The dose is determined by the amount needed to suppress muscle symptoms (fasciculations, twitching, and cramps). Based on reports from PALS and laboratory research, on average, a minimum of 16–18g of AAKG is required to have an effect. AAKG may cause diarrhea and bloating. Our experience has found that if you start with a low dose and gradually increase the dose not to exceed 18 grams over time these symptoms may be lessened or will stop. Do not take total dose at one time.

Deanna takes 18g of AAKG and divides it between breakfast, lunch and dinner. In addition, she takes 4, 300mg capsules of AKG every 1hr–1.5hrs between doses of AAKG up until bedtime. For the reasons stated above, if you need to increase the dose of AKG to decrease muscle symptoms, use AKG not AAKG. If you are very active, you may notice an increase in muscle symptoms. This means you have used up your energy supply and likely need more AKG.

Chapter Twenty-Three

GABA

Some of Deanna's symptoms, such as muscle rigidity and spasticity, could be caused by excessive glutamate, alone, or could be caused by a shortage of GABA, alone. Any imbalance of excitatory and inhibitory neurotransmitters can result in the muscle symptoms experienced by PALS. Magnetic resonance spectroscopy (MRS) has revealed both a shortage of GABA and an excess of glutamate in the brain of PALS compared to healthy people.[46]

The authors have heard from other people who do not have neurodegenerative diseases who claim that GABA calms them down, when they are anxious or under a lot of stress. The authors are not promoting GABA for this purpose. A balance of excitatory and inhibitory neurotransmitters is necessary in the body. Artificially adding one or the other can throw the body out of balance. In PALS, their bodies are already out of balance; therefore, it is necessary to add GABA to the diet to rebalance the excitatory and inhibitory neurotransmitters in PALS.

Adrenalin is an excitatory neurotransmitter, and Deanna experienced the effects of excess adrenalin and shortage of GABA when her muscles would become rigid.

---

46 http://www.alzforum.org/news/research-news/brain-imaging-suggests-neurotransmitter-imbalance-als.

This led to panic, more adrenalin, and even more muscle rigidity. Eventually, Deanna became an unbalanced human statue, causing her to fall like a tree, unable to even catch herself. Her muscles became entirely rigid, and fighting it only made the situation worse. Deanna's panic came from a loss of control over her own muscles. Taking GABA gave Deanna back her control.

A neurologist suggested a prescription drug by the name of Baclofen® for some of Deanna's symptoms. Upon researching Baclofen®, the authors found out that it is a form of GABA with an added radical. According to the literature, the extra radical supposedly allows the drug to pass through the blood brain barrier (BBB). The BBB is a layer of tightly packed cells that make up the walls of brain capillaries and prevent substances in the blood from diffusing freely into the brain. Passage across the cell membranes is determined by solubility in the lipid bilayer or recognition by a transport molecule.

GABA is a readily available nutritional supplement. However, some believe that GABA cannot pass the BBB. If a substance does *not* pass the BBB, the substance, when absorbed into the body, will not get to the brain. If a substance *does* pass the BBB, it may pass to the brain. Because Baclofen® is a form of GABA, the authors decided to have Deanna try GABA, first.

GABA has a long history of safe use as a dietary supplement, is naturally found in the body, and is inexpensive. When Deanna started taking GABA, she immediately noticed that she could carry a glass of water without shaking and spilling it. She could not do this before taking GABA. The change was truly remarkable. GABA reduced Deanna's spasticity and eliminated the human statue episodes that so unnerved Deanna.

It is recognized that spinal motor neurons extend beyond the blood brain barrier.[47] This may allow these motor neurons to be accessible to therapies that are not feasible for other neurons. The authors believe that GABA might somehow pass through the BBB and does get to the brain, but can't point to any evidence of this, other than Deanna's remarkable story. While the mechanism for delivery of GABA to the motor neurons is uncertain. Deanna's muscle spasticity improved after taking GABA. Deanna would not have improved, if GABA could not get to where it was needed. There is no denying this. Many PALS have reported similar results.

Perhaps, when a person has ALS, the GABA reaches only those motor neurons in the spinal cord that extend beyond the BBB, or perhaps the BBB of ALS patients doesn't function normally. Scientists might not know as much about the BBB and how it functions as they think. Regardless, GABA is an essential nutrient for ALS patients.

The GABA used by Deanna is an over the counter, sustained-release form that is absorbed in the intestine. This GABA seems to work well. The authors have heard that other forms of GABA do not work at all. So, it is

---

47   https://grants.nih.gov/grants/guide/rfa-files/RFA-NS-04-003. html; The etiology, pathogenesis and treatment of ALS; August 8, 2003; RFA-NS-04-003.

important to pay attention to the type of GABA you're using or prescribing for PALS. Dose changes according to the degree of spasticity and tremors present in the individual with ALS. Deanna takes 250 mg 2 times per day. If she feels more spastic, she increases the dose.

IMPORTANT: USE A SUSTAINED-RELEASE FORM OF GABA THAT IS ABSORBED IN THE INTESTINE. OTHER SOURCES OF GABA MAY BREAK DOWN BEFORE BEING ABSORBED.

Chapter Twenty-Four

Ubiquinol & NADH

If you look at the chart of the energy cycle, below, you will see that the part of the energy cycle utilizing AKG also needs NADH.

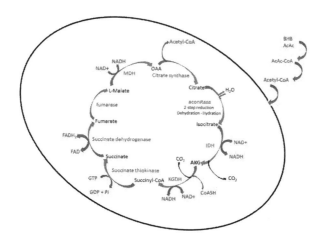

NADH is important in several reactions and is used with coenzyme Q10, also referred to as CoQ10. NADH is not absorbed by the body when ingested orally. So, the Deanna Protocol® recommends taking precursors for NADH, which are niacin and 5-hydroxytryptophan. Both niacin and 5-hydroxytryptophan are both well absorbed via oral administration. If the body has sufficient niacin and 5-hydroxytryptophan, it should be able to create enough NADH. NADH is essential in several of the reactions shown in the energy cycle, above. Coenzyme Q10, a fat soluble coenzyme, is also important in transporting electrons through an electron transport chain.

Electrons from NADH and succinate pass through the electron transport chain, thanks to CoQ10, which is capable of transporting electrons through the inner membrane of the mitochondria. The transport of electrons pumps protons (H+) across the membrane, which is used by ATP synthase to generate ATP. In the electron transport chain, CoQ10 is the electron carrier from enzyme complex I and enzyme complex II to enzyme complex III. CoQ10 was thought to be alone in its ability to transport electrons, but now scientists believe that vitamin K can substitute for CoQ10.[48] The authors suggest K2 for PALS and patients suffering from Parkinson's; however, this may be obtained from diet.

CoQ10 is produced by the human body in a complex system requiring proper functioning of several genes but is available, also, as a dietary supplement. CoQ10 is an essential coenzyme in the energy cycle[49] and has been

---

48   Bhalerao, S. and Clandinin,T.R. (2012). Vitamin K2 Takes Charge. *Science*, 336, 241-1242; and Vos, M., et al. (2012). *Science*, 336, 1306–1310.

49   Ernster, L; Dallner, G. (1995). Biochemical, physiological and medical aspects of ubiquinone function. *Biochimica et Biophysica Acta*, 1271.1, 195–204; and Dutton, P.L.; Ohnishi, T., Darrouzet, E., Leonard, M.A., Sharp, R.E., Cibney, B.R., Daldal, F. Moser, C.C. (2000). Coenzyme Q oxidation reduction reactions in mitochondrial electron transport. Kagan, V.E., Quinn, PJ. *Coenzyme Q: Molecular*

shown to be safe at dosages recommended in the Deanna Protocol®.[50] It is very important in muscle health, particularly.[51] Therefore, it is a reasonable dietary supplement for PALS suffering from muscle atrophy, when trying to improve muscle tone and muscle mass in PALS. CoQ10 in its reduced state is known as Ubiquinol.

The authors believe that the energy cycle is impaired in PALS, at least in those cells prematurely dying in PALS. CoQ10 can be taken safely[52] and is known to be essential to the energy cycle in cells. There is no direct evidence that any particular form of ALS is caused by a dysfunction in the supply of CoQ10 or NADH. There is no direct evidence that these substances benefit PALS. The reason for including them in the diet of PALS is to avoid any shortage of these essential substances, particularly when these substances are known to be important in the metabolism of AKG and the energy cycle in mitochondria. When dealing with a deadly disease that robs the muscles of strength and

---

mechanisms in health and disease, Boca Raton: CRC Press. pp. 65–82 (2000).

50 Hyson HC, Kieburtz K, Shoulson I, et al. (2010). Safety and tolerability of high-dosage coenzyme Q10 in Huntington's disease and healthy subjects. *Mov. Disord.*, 25.12, 1924–8.

51 Montero R, Sánchez-Alcázar J.A., Briones P., et al. (2008). Analysis of coenzyme Q10 in muscle and fibroblasts for the diagnosis of CoQ10 deficiency syndromes. *Clin. Biochem*, 41.9, 697–700; and Trevisson E., Dimauro S., Navas P., Salviati L. (2011). Coenzyme Q deficiency in muscle. *Curr. Opin. Neurol.*, 24.5, 449–56.

52 Hathcock J.N., Shao A. (2006). Risk assessment for coenzyme Q10 (Ubiquinone). *Regul. Toxicol. Pharmacol.* 45.3 282–8.

results in muscle atrophy, why not do all that you can to support nerve and muscle health?

Ubiquinol and the precursors for NADH are readily available and not expensive. If some cell death in PALS is preventable by oral administration of Ubiquinol and precursors for NADH, then supplementation makes sense. PALS really can't risk cell death or cellular inactivity from lack of these essential factors. The Deanna Protocol® recommends taking Ubiquinol as a source of CoQ10 and niacin and 5-hydroxytryptophan to support production of NADH. By supplementing the diets of PALS with CoQ10, niacin and 5-hydroxytryptophan, the energy cycle in cells is supported.

Ubiquinol is a more potent form of CoQ10. The most effective form Idebenone has been taken off the market. Thus, it is unavailable, except by prescription and very expensive. Laboratory data suggests taking 1,000mg – 1,400mg of Ubiquinol daily. If a more effective form, such as Idebenone is used less may be required.

NADH is not readily absorbed by the GI system, which is why the Deanna Protocol® includes niacin, a precursor to NADH, which can be absorbed by the GI system. Another precursor to NADH is 5-hydroxytryptophane [5-HTP] and is also absorbed. Care must be taken, and these supplements should only be taken after AAKG and GABA are having the desired effect on muscle symptoms.

NIACIN AND 5-HYDROXYTRYPTOPHANE ARE RECOMMENDED SUPPLEMENTS SUPPORTING THE DEANNA PROTOCOL®. BUT THIS COULD

CHANGE IF PRELIMINARY RESEARCH IN CELL MODELS IS CONFIRMED IN PALS OR SOD1 MICE MODELS. UBIQUINOL IS RECOMMENDED IN THE DEANNA PROTOCOL®. CAUTION: EXCESS UBIQUINOL, NIACIN AND 5-HYDROXYTRYTOPHANE CAN BE TOXIC TO THE LIVER AND MOTOR NEURONS. DO NOT TAKE THESE SUPPLEMENTS WITHOUT CONSULTING YOUR PHYSICIAN. THE DEANNA PROTOCOL® IS A WORK IN PROGRESS.

Chapter Twenty-Five

Arginine

Excess extracellular glutamate can kill adjacent cells by altering the normal calcium channels, causing sodium ions (Na+) and fluid to flood the cells. Distention and, ultimately, rupture of the cellular membrane can result, releasing more glutamate into the extracellular space. This is a mechanism that could cause cascading motor neuron death affecting region after region in PALS. Arginine might have a positive effect.

One person taking the Deanna Protocol® mistakenly took arginine aspartate instead of arginine-AKG. Nevertheless, this patient's muscle symptoms improved, somewhat. Another person took arginine-AKG with a ratio of 2 arginine to 1 AKG. The authors were concerned that the nitric oxide response from taking so much arginine could cause some complications, if the dose of arginine was too high. I recommended a change to the type of arginine-AKG, changing the ratio from 2 to 1 arginine down to 1 to 1 arginine, lowering the level of arginine. However, he reported feeling better on the arginine-AKG with a 2 to 1 ratio and changed back. In both instances, more arginine was beneficial.

We know that glutamate is removed from the brain via the blood vessels that are in contact with the brain tissue.

Nitric acid increases with an increase in arginine. Nitric acid causes vasodilation, an increase in the diameter of blood vessels, increasing blood flow through the blood vessels. Perhaps, vasodilation allows more glutamate to be removed from the brain. This reasoning could be questioned by researchers, because there is no direct evidence of this mechanism in humans. However, this mechanism has been proven in mice.[53] The Deanna Protocol® includes arginine as part of the arginine-AKG (AAKG) taken to provide cells with energy. Care must be taken not to take too much arginine and to monitor any conditions that might be exacerbated by vasodilation. Arginine at the levels provided by the Deanna Protocol® is within safe limits. Therefore, arginine is an important part of the Deanna Protocol®. However, care should be taken to consult a physician before taking arginine.

According to Boston University's Center for the Study of Traumatic Encephalopathy, in closed head trauma,

---

53   Ghadge, G.D., Slusher, B., Bodner A., D al Canto, M., Wozniak, K,. Thomas, A., et al (2003). Glutamate Carboxypeptidase II Inhibition Protects Motor Neurons from Death in Familial Amyotrophic Lateral Sclerosis Models. *Proceedings of the National Academy of Science USA*, 100.16, 9554–9559. http://www.pnas.org/content/100/16/9554; Rothstein, J., Sarjubhai, P., Melissa, R., Haenggeli, C., Huang, Y., Bergles, D. ... Fisher, P.B. (2005). Beta-lactam Antibiotics Offer Neuroprotection By Increasing Glutamate Transporter Expression. *Nature*, 433.7021, 73–77. http://dx.doi.org/10.1038/nature03180; Perez-Mato, M, Ramos-Cabrer, P, Sobrino, T., Blanco, M., Ruban, A., Mirelman, D., Menendez, P., Castillo, J., Campos, F. (2014). Human recombinant glutamate oxaloacetate transaminase 1 (GOT1) supplemented with oxaloacetate induces a protective effect after cerebral ischemia. *Cell Death and Disease*, 5, e992. http://dx.doi.org/10.1038/cddis.2013.507.

concussions, and strokes, nerve cells die in a localized area. These cells release glutamate into the extracellular space. The glutamate then causes surrounding cells to die. This same mechanism might be occurring in patients with neurodegenerative diseases, such as ALS, Alzheimer's and Parkinson's. To limit effects of injury, patients should be treated to neutralize or remove excess glutamate.[54] Until GOT becomes available for human consumption, the vasodilation caused by arginine intake might be the best option that PALS have.

THE DEANNA PROTOCOL® RECOMMENDS ARGININE-AKG AS A SOURCE OF AKG, WHICH PROVIDES LEVELS OF ARGININE GENERALLY REGARDED AS SAFE. MORE THAN 18 GRAMS OF ARGININE PER DAY COULD BE HARMFUL OR DANGEROUS TO YOUR HEALTH. USE A SOURCE OF AAKG WITH 1:1 ARGININE TO AKG.

---

54 Redler R.L., & Dokholyan, N.V. (2012). The complex molecular biology of amyotrophic lateral sclerosis (ALS). *Prog Mol Biol Transl Sci.* 107, 215–62. http://www.sciencedirect.com/science/article/pii/B9780123858832000023.

Chapter Twenty-Six

Coconut Oil

Dr. Mary Newport is an intelligent and accomplished physician. She is an author of a book related to her experiences in treating her husband's Alzheimer's. Her book is entitled, *Alzheimer's Disease: What If There Were a Cure?* Dr. Newport used coconut oil to treat her husband and noticed significant improvement in his cognitive function and physical mobility as a result. As it turns out, coconut oil also feeds the energy cycle in the mitochondria. Coconut oil contains caprylic acid, which is a medium chain triglyceride[55] that breaks down to ketone bodies, which contribute to the energy cycle. Let's take a second look at the mitochondria and the energy cycle.

Acetyl-CoA is shown as entering the mitochondria organelle. This Acetyl-CoA feeds the energy cycle and is produced by the metabolizing in the liver of the medium chain triglycerides. Medium Chain Triglycerides (MCTs) and the ketogenic diet also create ketone bodies that feed the energy cycle. For example, these ketone bodies are B-H-B and AcAc, which might act, also, as cogs in the gears of the energy cycle, perhaps, helping an inefficient

---

55   Medium chain triglycerides are molecules that are easily absorbed through the skin by the body due to their small size, unlike long chain triglycerides.

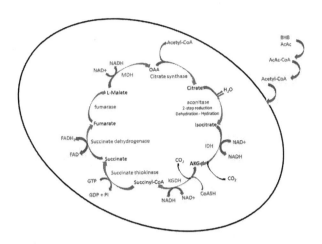

energy cycle to prevent cell death in PALS and patients with other neurodegenerative diseases. The top right of the diagram, above, shows BHB and AcAc, ketone bodies, being metabolized. For example, AcAc may be metabolized to AcAc-CoA, which is metabolized further to Acetyl-CoA, which provides energy in the energy cycle.

Ketone bodies and ketones are distinct substances, despite the similar names. In this diagram, AKG, a ketone, is depicted at the lower right side of the energy cycle, within the mitochondria. Presumably, the metabolizing of BHB and AcAc occur elsewhere than in the mitochondria. Yet, these ketone bodies do enter into the energy cycle. Exactly how the ketone bodies enter into the energy cycle is an important piece of information that, to my knowledge, is lacking.

Ketone bodies [KB] may be derived from coconut oil, a ketogenic diet and medium chain triglycerides [MCT].

KB's might come into the energy cycle at a different point or points than AKG. The ketone, AKG, is found within the cell. KB's are formed in the liver by the breakdown of MCT's such as coconut oil (caprylic acid) or a ketogenic diet. Then, the KB's or metabolites of KB's migrate to cells and enter the energy cycle.

The point at which the ketone bodies enter the energy cycle is debated. Some say it is before AKG. Others say it is after AKG. It could be both. Studies sponsored by Winning the Fight, Inc. at USF used ALS mice to compare the effects of a ketogenic diet and the Deanna Protocol® with control SOD1-G93A mice fed a regular diet.[56] The mice on the Deanna Protocol® lived more than 7.5% longer, after the onset of disease, than control mice. This research confirms the observations from Deanna and other PALS who have adopted the Deanna Protocol®. Deanna did not benefit from the ketogenic diet the way that she has benefitted from the Deanna Protocol®. Whether this is due to the limited amount of energy provided by a ketogenic diet to the cells or other reasons is something that could be explored, if more resources were available.

The energy cycle, a chain of chemical reactions, produces energy via the creation of high energy phosphate

---

56 Csilla Ari, Angela M. Poff, Heather E. Held, Carol S. Landon, Craig R. Goldhagen, Nicholas Mavromates, Dominic P. D'Agostino, "Metabolic Therapy with Deanna Protocol Supplementation Delays Disease Progression and Extends Survival in Amyotrophic Lateral Sclerosis (ALS) Mouse Model," *Plos One*, (July 25, 2014); see http://dx.plos.org/10.1371/journal.pone.0103526.

bonds. Each phase in the cycle is a chemical reaction that uses different substances to produce a high energy phosphate bond. The way that the authors envision this is that, when every single reaction in the cycle creates an energy bond, the cycle produces more than enough energy for a cell. However, when there is a break down in the cycle caused by a failure in just one chemical reaction, the rest of the chemical reactions that should follow don't occur. No more energy bonds are created. In this case, the cycle might not create sufficient energy in a cell, and the cell dies, prematurely.

If this hypothesis is true, then failed chemical reactions occurring earlier in the cycle have a greater impact on the final energy produced. More reactions follow, depending on the earlier reactions to provide the molecule that should be used in a later step. If ALS is a metabolic disease, and a reaction providing AKG is to blame, then providing AKG in the diet might allow the reactions to continue. This can only occur if AKG can find its way to the mitochondria. Whether or not this is possible is a subject of debate. But the evidence from the study with SOD1-G93A mice, Deanna's results and reports from PALS around the world is persuasive evidence that, somehow, AKG finds its way to the mitochondria. If this occurs, then the energy cycle in the mitochondria begins, again, with the AKG step in the lower right of the drawing, above. However, the subject matter is so complex that designing a test of this hypothesis is not easy. Much more work needs to be done to determine how ALS derails the energy cycle in cells. The study conducted at USF showed that only the mice treated with the Deanna Protocol® still had mitochondria visible in motor neurons on electron microscopy. The motor neurons of mice fed a standard diet and those on a ketogenic diet lacked mitochondria.[57]

One interesting hypothesis is that AKG may selectively enter those cells distressed by a lack of energy. Some research suggests that the polarity of cells may change during the initial phases of programmed cell death, called apoptosis. The complex changes that occur in a cell during apoptosis might allow AKG to enter those cells, while healthy cells prevent AKG from entering. If AKG enters only those cells in distress and reverses the process of apoptosis, before permanent damage is done, then AKG could be highly selective and much more potent than ketone bodies, which presumably are available to all cells, those operating normally and those in distress. If true, taking AKG selectively revives those cells in distress, while KB's resulting from a ketogenic diet or MCT's are not selective. This hypothesis explains why AKG works at all and why it would work better than KB's derived from sources such as coconut oil. By selectively targeting cells in distress, then, AKG could have a much greater impact compared to KB's,

---

57   Csilla Ari, Angela M. Poff, Heather E. Held, Carol S. Landon, Craig R. Goldhagen, Nicholas Mavromates, Dominic P. D'Agostino, "Metabolic Therapy with Deanna Protocol Supplementation Delays Disease Progression and Extends Survival in Amyotrophic Lateral Sclerosis (ALS) Mouse Model," *Plos One*, (July 25, 2014); see http://dx.plos.org/10.1371/journal.pone.0103526.

which are spread thinner by being taken up by healthy cells and cells in distress, equally.

The Deanna Protocol® includes massage with coconut oil, because massage allows the MCT's in coconut oil to be absorbed through the skin and to directly affect atrophied muscles. There is some evidence that massage with coconut oil improves muscle tone and helps in recovery of some of the strength in the muscles lost due to the ravages of ALS. Whether this is due to the MCT's in coconut oil is not known, but massage with coconut oil does not harm PALS. So, if there is evidence of any benefit, then why not continue? On Winning the Fight's forum, www.winningthefight.org, the authors encountered Butch Machlin, who lives in Mexico City. Butch's results were remarkable. By massaging coconut oil into his very weak and atrophied thigh muscle, Butch's thigh muscle gained three inches in circumference, as measured by his physical therapist.

Coconut oil contains Caprylic acid, a medium chain triglyceride. Medium chain triglycerides are molecules that are small enough to be absorbed right through all the skin's layers and into the muscles below.[58] According to Dr. Mary Newport, Caprylic acid goes straight into the mitochondria of muscle cells[59] and helps them produce

---

58   Björntorp, P. (1968). Rates of Oxidation of Different Fatty Acids by Isolated Rat Liver Mitochondria. *The Journal of Biological Chemistry*, 243, 2130–2133. http://www.jbc.org/content/243/9/2130.short.

59   Mitochondria are the part of a cell responsible for producing energy to keep the cells alive and functioning.

energy. The mitochondria in the muscle cells near the myo-neuro junction[60] of neurodegenerative cells are depolarized.[61] When this depolarization occurs, the electrical charge needed to stimulate energy production in the mitochondria no longer exists. When mitochondria stop producing energy in the cells, the cells die, the muscle cells are unable to contract, causing atrophy. Adding Caprylic acid via topical coconut oil treatment prevents cell death and prevents muscle atrophy. For Butch Machlin and other PALS, coconut oil massage actually allows the patient to regain muscle mass. This is why our program also focuses on treating the muscles directly by massaging them with coconut oil. In Deanna's experience, ingesting coconut oil orally does *not* provide the same benefit.

MASSAGING MUSCLES WITH COCONUT OIL DAILY, OR MORE OFTEN, IF POSSIBLE, IS A RECOMMENDED PRACTICE IN THE DEANNA PROTOCOL®.

---

60   The myo-neuro junction is where the nerve connects to the muscle.

61   Turner, N., Hariharan, K., TidAng, J., et al., (2009). Enhancement of muscle mitochondrial oxidative capacity and alterations in insulin action are lipid species dependent: potent tissue-specific effects of medium-chain fatty acids. *Diabetes*, 48, 2547–2554.

Chapter Twenty-Seven

Non-exhausting Exercise

The ALS diagnosis is usually made when physicians notice extreme muscle atrophy.[62] The diagnosis takes too long. On average, ALS patients typically note that their ALS symptoms first started about two years before a diagnosis of ALS is made. The issue of muscle weakness and atrophy brought me to investigate the idea of exercise, which is now an important component of the Deanna Protocol®.

Many years ago, Dr. Tedone gained insight from a friend and little did he know that his insight would help his daughter, Deanna. Jack Castiglia, who suffered from the effects of polio since childhood, became a nationally renowned expert in joint and limb bracing. He told Dr. Tedone of a method for treating polio that was developed in Australia by Sister Kenny.[63] Her method for treating polio had far more success than the typical method used in the United States. In the United States, polio patients were treated by immobilizing the affected muscles until the pain subsided. The affected limbs were then placed on passive

62   http://www.hopkinsmedicine.org/neurology_neurosurgery/specialty_areas/als/conditions/als_amyotrophic_lateral_sclerosis.html.

63   Kenny, E. & Ostenso, M., (1943). *And They Shall Walk*. Bruce Publishing Co, Minneapolis-St Paul.

assisted range of motion exercises.[64] This treatment would almost always result in paralysis of the affected limbs.

Sister Kenny never immobilized affected muscles and limbs. Instead of *passive* assisted range of motion exercises, she used hydrotherapy and *active* assisted range of motion exercises.[65] She began this therapy as soon as polio was diagnosed. Coupled with the knowledge that ALS is diagnosed due to severe atrophy about two years after onset, the authors questioned the currently accepted belief that ALS patients should do minimal exercise. Remember to challenge the status quo, and do what is necessary, even if unconventional.

Muscle atrophy is caused by inactivity of affected muscles. Perhaps, muscles are inactive, because patients find it hard to move their muscles due to a lack of nerve stimulation. In addition, PALS are told don't exercise or only exercise with passive range of motion exercises! Based on Sister Kenny's success with active assisted range of motion exercise, the authors developed a hypothesis. The hypothesis is that there is a retrograde stimulus present in polio patients and PALS.

Ordinarily, nerve stimulation causes a muscle to be stimulated. By retrograde stimulus, the authors mean that muscle stimulation causes corresponding nerves to

---

64   Passive assisted range of motion exercises are exercises in which a therapist or a machine moves the limb, requiring no effort from the patient.

65   Active assisted range of motion exercises are exercises requiring patients to exert effort to move their own muscles.

be stimulated. Deanna was suffering from muscle atrophy. So, she began an exercise regimen that would stimulate her muscles using active range of motion exercises. She hoped that this would induce a retrograde stimulation of nerve cells and improve her muscle tone. She used a Power Plate,[66] which stimulates the stretch reflex. Also, she performed progressive resistive exercises, aerobic exercises, breathing exercises, hand exercises, speech exercises, and stretching. Six-plus years into the disease, Deanna's muscle atrophy is limited.

Retrograde stimulation is not a widely accepted hypothesis for patients with motor neuron diseases. However, the importance of muscle stimulation in reinnervation is widely supported in recent research.

ALS, polio and trauma can kill motor neurons. It is very well known that it is the death of motor neurons that denervates muscles in each of these.[67] The death of some but not all motor neurons in a pool of motor neurons leads to the sprouting of intact axons within the muscle to

---

66 Power Plate is a brand of exercise device with an oscillating platform on which one stands to perform exercises. The oscillations excite the stretch reflexes in the muscles which increase the tone, often more quickly than if exercise were performed on a stable platform. The Power Plate is used by professional athletes.

67 Sharrard, W.J. (1955). The distribution of the permanent paralysis in the lower limb in poliomyelitis; a clinical and pathological study. *J Bone Joint Surg. Br.* 37-B, 540–558; Tandan, R. and Bradley, W.G. (1985). Amyotrophic lateral sclerosis: Part 1. Clinical features, pathology, and ethical issues in management. *Ann. Neurol.* 18, 271–280; and Thomas, C.K. (1997). Contractile properties of human thenar muscles paralyzed by spinal cord injury. *Muscle Nerve* 20, 788–799.

reinnervate the muscle.[68] Death of all of motor neurons in a pool of motor neurons denervates the muscle completely, causing rapid and progressive atrophy.[69] However, stimulation of denervated muscles reduces muscle atrophy.[70] Research has shown that the effects of stimulation are local.[71] After denervation, it has been observed that acetylcholine receptors become expressed along muscle fiber

68 Thompson, W. and Jansen, J.K. (1977). The extent of sprouting of remaining motor units in partly denervated immature and adult rat soleus muscle. *Neuroscience*, 2, 523–535.

69 Degens, H., Kosar, S.N., Hopman, M.T., and de Haan, A. (2008). The time course of denervation-induced changes is similar in soleus muscles of adult and old rats. *Applied Physiology, Nutrition, and Metabolism* 33, 299–308; and Finkelstein, D.I., Dooley, P.C., and Luff, A.R. (1993). Recovery of muscle after different periods of denervation and treatments. *Muscle Nerve* 16, 769–777.

70 Hennig, R. and Lømo, T. (1987). Effects of chronic stimulation on the size and speed of long-term denervated and innervated rat fast and slow skeletal muscles. *Acta Physiol. Scand.* 130, 115–131; Salmons, S. and Vrbova, G. (1969). The influence of activity on some contractile characteristics of mammalian fast and slow muscles. *J Physiol.* 201, 535–549; and Westgaard, R.H. and Lomo, T. (1988). Control of contractile properties within adaptive ranges by patterns of impulse activity in the rat. *J Neurosci.* 8, 4415–4426.

71 Mödlin, M., Forstner, C., Hofer, C., Mayr, W., Richter, W., Carraro, U., Protasi, F., and Kern, H. (2005). Electrical stimulation of denervated muscles: first results of a clinical study. *Artif. Organs* 29, 203–206.; M., Forstner, C., Hofer, C., Mayr, W., Richter, W., Carraro, U., Protasi, F., and Kern, H. (2005). Electrical stimulation of denervated muscles: first results of a clinical study. *Artif. Organs* 29, 203–206; M., Forstner, C., Hofer, C., Mayr, W., Richter, W., Carraro, U., Protasi, F., and Kern, H. (2005). Electrical stimulation of denervated muscles: first results of a clinical study. *Artif. Organs* 29, 203–206.

membranes.[72] The reclustering of acetylcholine receptors is a critical step in the reinnervation of functional muscles, and it is known that acetylcholine receptors can be reclustered by direct electrical stimulation of the muscle tissues.[73] Therefore, it is well established that muscle stimulation is a critical step in reinnervation of functional muscle tissue, and the authors believe that non-exhaustive exercises can be effective in providing a type of retrograde stimulus that helps to reinnervate the muscles. The opposite point of view, to avoid exercise, which is the position of most of the neurological community in the U.S., will inevitably lead to muscle atrophy and death of the muscle tissue and of the motor neurons.

NON-FATIGUING EXERCISE IS RECOMMENDED AS AN IMPORTANT PART OF THE DEANNA PROTOCOL®.

---

72   Tsay, H.J. and Schmidt, J. (1989). Skeletal muscle denervation activates acetylcholine receptor genes. *J Cell Biol.* 108, 1523–1526.

73   Goldman, D., Brenner, H.R., and Heinemann, S. (1988). Acetylcholine receptor alpha-, beta-, gamma-, and delta-subunit mRNA levels are regulated by muscle activity. *Neuron* 1, 329–333; and Lømo, T. and Westgaard, R.H. (1975). Further studies on the control of ACh sensitivity by muscle activity in the rat. *J Physiol.* 252, 603–626.

Chapter Twenty-Eight

Chelation

Chelation is a treatment used to remove heavy metals from the circulatory system. Deanna underwent chelation treatments without much to show for it. Some studies have shown no benefit from chelation therapy.[74] However, Deanna came to believe that toxic metals in the Chinese drywall in her house could have been the trigger for her ALS. The authors thought that removing the heavy metals might be a way of stopping the disease. So, Deanna started a chelation treatment to try to remove strontium and other heavy metals from her tissues.

A high school friend of Dr. Tedone, introduced him to Dr. Benjamin Brooks a neurologist and head of the ALS/MDA Center in Charlotte, North Carolina. He told Dr. Tedone that he agreed with everything that Deanna was doing, except chelation treatments. Dr. Brooks emphasized that heavy metal deposits in tissues like fat will not do any damage, but when removed from benign tissue, the metals can begin to circulate in the body. Then, the heavy metals could be deposited in more important tissues, such as muscle cells or nerve cells. A study showed that this was

---

74 Praline J, Guennoc A M, Limousin N, Hallak H, de Toffol B, Corcia P. (2007). ALS and mercury intoxication: a relationship? *Clin Neurol Neurosurg*, 109.10, 880–3.

more than a possibility.[75] Dr. Brooks' agreement with the Deanna Protocol® treatment at least provided some peace of mind that she was on the right track, but the authors still worry that chelation might have caused more harm than good in Deanna's case. By the time that Dr. Brooks was consulted, Deanna had been on a chelation treatment for a year, without any positive results. She stopped chelation.

CHELATION IS **NOT** RECOMMENDED FOR PALS AND IS NOT PART OF THE DEANNA PROTOCOL®.

---

75   Ewan K, Pamphlett R. (1996). Increased inorganic mercury in spinal motor neurons following chelating agents. *Neurotoxicology*, 17, 343–349.

Chapter Twenty-Nine

Ketogenic Diet

Deanna was on a ketogenic diet (KD) and taking oral coconut oil. Also, she tried substances that would boost ketone bodies. There was some anecdotal evidence that KD could help PALS, but KD was a difficult regimen for Deanna. Dr. Tedone realized that KD was designed to increase ketone levels in the body, and AKG is a ketone. He hypothesized that AKG should be able to achieve the same goal. Having studied the break down products of glutamate, Dr. Tedone knew that AKG was one of the substances produced when glutamate is metabolized. So, logically, if glutamate is *not broken down*, the body must *lack sufficient AKG*. The logic seems undeniable, now, but nobody was looking in this direction. It took time, precious time, for Dr. Tedone to piece all of this together.

Deanna started taking AKG and, very shortly afterward, she was able to roll over in bed, normally, which she had been unable to do for quite some time. The KD regimen had not helped. Nothing else had helped the muscle fatigue and weakness. The AKG was the first substance that noticeably helped Deanna regain some of her strength. At that time, she was taking oral coconut oil, Tamoxifen and Axona®, while trying to comply with the KD. None of these were doing anything for her, so Deanna discontinued all of them. The AKG was working. At one point, Deanna ran out of AKG and her muscle symptoms increased markedly within a day, only to subside quickly when she resumed the AKG.

THE KD DID NOT WORK FOR DEANNA OR IN SOD1-G93A MICE. WE DO NOT RECOMMEND THIS FOR ALS.

Chapter Thirty

Stem Cell Therapy

Stem cell therapies hold promise, but the authors are still waiting to see if the therapies are both safe and effective. Stem cell treatments are not benign. Usually, stem cells are placed in the cerebral spinal fluid either by injection or by laminectomy of the cervical or lumbar spine.

Recent research at Hadassah University Medical Center in Jerusalem and Mayo Clinic in Minnesota has treated a single patient with ALS and myasthenia gravis (MG), another muscular disease. A news article from January 2014 summarizes the research.[76] The actual research paper describes it in length and was published in the February 2014 issue of *Muscle and Nerve*.[77] This is

---

76 http://www.medicaldaily.com/als-patient-improves-nurown-new-stem-cell-therapy-company-awaits-fda-decision-phase-ii-trial-266380. *"...technology that stimulates autologous bone marrow-derived Mesenchymal Stem Cells (MSCs) to secrete Neurotropic Factors (NTF). This means that a patient's own stem cells are removed and then engineered to create specialized neuron-supporting cells; after this, they are transplanted back into the patient's own body at or near the site of damage, for instance, directly into the patient's spine or muscles. Because it uses an individual's own stem cells, this treatment is considered relatively safe..."*

77 http://onlinelibrary.wiley.com/doi/10.1002/mus.24143/abstract. *"...both cognitive and motor disabilities improved after the initial course*

very encouraging, again, if proven both safe and effective.

Stem cell therapy can also involve hormones. There are naturally occurring hormones that are reproduced synthetically and that have been used for years to reconstitute the bone marrow treated with radiation for cancer. These are Neupogen® [G-CSF] and Leukine [GM-CSF]. These hormones stimulate the bone marrow to form stem cells which then are expected to become new healthy nerve cells, and thus, repair the nervous system. There is a hematologist on the east coast of Florida who offers a six-week treatment with Neupogen® for $50,000. He claims to have had success with stroke and Parkinson's patients and was willing to treat Deanna.

The authors have reviewed both publicly available and proprietary research on this type of treatment for ALS and remain unconvinced that the treatment could work without nutritional support such as the Deanna Protocol® provides. A clinical trial pairing the Deanna Protocol® with this type of treatment intrigues the authors, but none of the drug companies have yet agreed to combine the Deanna Protocol® with a clinical trial of their drug. The authors do not believe that the science supports the effectiveness of these drugs for the treatment of ALS without the Deanna Protocol®.

Deanna tried Neupogen®. It is very expensive and entails daily subcutaneous injections. Deanna responded

---

of cell therapy; these benefits were reversed over the following months... repeated transplantation might be needed to maintain and enhance the clinical benefits of stem cell therapies in neurological diseases."

with extreme fatigue and no improvement. She discontinued Neupogen®. Deanna switched to Leukine but had an allergic reaction. This too was discontinued. So, neither drug worked for Deanna.

Dr. Tedone still believes a valid approach is to remove whatever is making cells die and to combine this treatment with autologous stem cell therapy or nerve growth factors derived from autologous stem cells. Even Neupogen® might be a valid approach, but dosage and frequency would need to be managed. Deanna's negative reaction could have been the result of the wrong dosage or frequency, but until pre-clinical research and a clinical trial pin these down, Deanna will not try it again.

An ALS patient contacted me to tell me he was offered the last place in a clinical trial using this hormone on 12 ALS patients. I never tell an individual with ALS/ND what to do but I give them the information they need and refer them to their treating physicians. I had been given the proprietary research done on this hormone in every country but the US. All reports were equivocal. Some PALS initially got better, but then their disease progressed again after a short while. I called the neurologist running this trial and told him that the research he was doing had already been done. He said he knew that. Why was he repeating it? The cost was $5,000 per patient for the hormone, *not* including overhead and salaries, so this was a very expensive study, not funded by a pharmaceutical company but funded by charitable donations. I told this neurologist that we could probably get the pharmaceutical company to fund a trial using the hormone in conjunction with the DP. I told him I would talk to the pharmaceutical company and get back to him. I called him several times but he never returned my calls. So a lot of time and money was wasted and anguish was caused in these 12 PALS as he watched them deteriorate while taking a substance that the neurologist knew would not work. Why?

I read about another trial in a patient who had received stem cells into the cerebral spinal fluid. He also improved for a while, but then his disease progressed again. The physician's response to this was that the patient only received 50,000 stem cells and he implied that 5,000,000 stem cells would change the outcome. Why would anyone believe that adding even more stem cells to an environment that was killing cells would not also kill the new cells?

THE DEANNA PROTOCOL® DOES **NOT** RECOMMEND STEM CELL THERAPY AT THIS TIME, UNTIL IT IS PROVEN TO BE SAFE.

Chapter Thirty-One

Glutamate Oxaloacetate Transaminase

Recent research at the Weizmann Institute and the Dana Foundation[78] highlights this possible mechanism for ALS progression and gives hope that the progression can be stopped. When motor neurons die, glutamate accumulates in the extracellular space. A normal ratio of intracellular glutamate to extracellular glutamate is 10,000 to 1. If glutamate is released when cells die and the number of cells releasing glutamate is sufficient, then excess glutamate can build up in the extracellular space. If this happens, then glutamate in the extracellular space can rise to toxic levels, unless the body is able to remove glutamate from the extracellular space. A break down in the mechanism that removes excess glutamate could be a mechanism for spreading ALS from segment to segment, which is commonly observed in ALS patients.

Perhaps, in the beginning, ALS is limited to a few damaged cells; however, by the release of glutamate in the extracellular space, a cascade effect occurs that implicates surrounding cells. If this is the case, then dysfunctional

---

78 Teichberg, V., Vikhanski, L. (2007, May). Protecting the Brain from a Glutamate Storm. *The Dana Foundation*. Retrieved from http://www.dana.org/news/cerebrum/detail.aspx?id=7376.

gene and/or enzymes, locally, could lead to the death of motor neurons in a wider area. This cascade effect could cause the death of surrounding motor neurons, which release more glutamate into the extracellular space, affecting even more motor neurons, and so on.

In Alzheimer's, excess glutamate is found in all areas of the brain. In Parkinson's, excess glutamate occurs in the *substantia nigra*, which are black areas in the mid-brain containing dopamine-producing neurons. In ALS, excess glutamate is found in the brain, the brain stem or posterior columns of the spinal cord. The diversity of symptoms at the onset of ALS is indicative of the diverse locations where excess glutamate can be found. Different areas of the brain control different regions of the body and different aspects of the body's functionality. I believe that the symptoms first noticed by PALS correspond to the regions of the brain, brain stem or posterior column of the spinal cord first affected by death of motor neurons. The hypothesis that excess glutamate causes a cascade of neuron death is consistent with the evidence.

Research on mice at the Weizmann Institute reveals that there is a physiological mechanism to regulate the quantity of intracellular and extracellular glutamate. The normal 10,000 to 1 ratio of intracellular to extracellular glutamate is regulated by the body. When an extracellular concentration of glutamate becomes greater than a concentration of glutamate in endothelial cells that surround capillaries in contact with brain tissue, glutamate increases in these endothelial cells. The increased concentration in the endothelial cells causes more glutamate to enter into circulation in the blood, and the body of a normal person will remove the excess glutamate by metabolic processes in the liver and through excretion.

The authors have been in communication with Dr. Ruban of the Weizmann Institute. Dr. Ruban believes that the most effective way of removing glutamate from the circulatory system is by administering glutamate oxaloacetate transaminase (GOT). This has proven to be much more effective than use of oxaloacetate, alone, in studies done on ALS mice. (Based on personal communications with Dr. Ruban formerly of the Weizmann Institute.)] Oxaloacetate is used in the TCA cycle and only lasts 15 to 30 minutes in blood circulation. Clinical trials are currently planned to see if GOT has the same effect in humans that it does in ALS mice.[79] A safe source of GOT for human consumption is not yet available for PALS. On the other hand, oxaloacetate is available for human use, and the authors cautiously advise prescribing oxaloacetate for ALS patients, in an attempt to stop progression of the disease, until clinical trials for use of GOT show that it is safe and effective. Research suggests that blood glutamate scavengers should be effective in reducing glutamate

---

79   Ghadge G D, Slusher B., Bodner, A., D al Canto, M., Wozniak, K., Thomas, A., et al (2003). Glutamate Carboxypeptidase II Inhibition Protects Motor Neurons from Death in Familial Amyotrophic Lateral Sclerosis Models. *Proceedings of the National Academy of Science USA,* 100.16,   9554–9559.   http://www.pnas.org/content/100/16/9554;   and http://www.weizmann.ac.il/neurobiology/labs/teichberg/PDFs/Zlotnik-JNA2009.pdf.

levels in extracellular fluids, but it is unclear if oxaloace-
tate resides long enough in the blood to be effective.[80]
WE RECOMMEND PATIENCE UNTIL A SAFE
SOURCE OF GOT BECOMES AVAILABLE AND IS
TESTED FOR SAFETY AND EFFICACY IN CLINI-
CAL TRIALS. WINNING THE FIGHT IS TRYING
TO SPONSOR A CLINICAL TRIAL, COMBINING
GOT AND/OR OXALOACETATE AND THE DEANNA
PROTOCOL®. WHILE WE BELIEVE THAT OXALO-
ACETATE CAN BE SAFELY PRESCRIBED FOR USE
BY PALS, WE CAUTION PALS AND CAREGIVERS
TO CLOSELY MONITOR ITS USE UNDER A DOC-
TORS SUPERVISION. THE SHORT HALF-LIFE OF
OXALOACETATE IN THE BLOOD COULD LIMIT
ITS EFFECTIVENESS.

---

80   http://www.ncbi.nlm.nih.gov/pmc/articles/PMC3431845/.

Chapter Thirty-Two

Quick Reference

Everything taken in The Deana Protocol® is already found in a healthy person's body, and the purpose of the protocol is to provide those substances that are missing or needed in a greater quantity in PALS.

- Supplements include AAKG, AKG, and GABA.

SUPPLEMENT	DOSAGE	PURPOSE
AAKG	Begin with standard dosage on bottle and increase slowly to 18g/day or as needed to reduce symptoms.	Delivers energy to nerves
AKG	300 mg pills take approx. every hour (you are awake) between doses of AAKG. May be listed as alpha Keto-glutaric acid	Delivers energy to nerves
Tryptophan	50 mg 1x/day (take at PM with niacin)	5-hydroxy tryptophan is a precursor to NADH and also serotonin and melatonin, both inhibitory neuro-transmitters

GABA	Up to 250 mg 2x/day or as needed to reduce symptoms.	Inhibitory neuro-transmitter

- Antioxidants: Glutathione either intravenous or liposomal

  GSH is the most effective nervous system antioxidant known to man. The best delivery system of GSH is IV 3000 mg once a week. The dose is determined by what is currently used by neurologists and wellness clinics. GSH can be delivered by suppository, Liposomal GSH, and sustained release GSH (sold by Thorne Research). Deanna gets the IV and takes sustained release GSH. In recommending this, we have accepted a large amount of research indicating the effectiveness of GSH in neutralizing reactive oxygen species which are known to be detrimental to nerve cells.

- Massage with extra virgin coconut oil, which contains caprylic acid, which enhances energy production in the mitochondria of the muscle cells.

  Massage with extra virgin coconut oil. Anecdotal evidence reveals that muscle strength and size can be improved with this regimen. We have anecdotal evidence that massage with coconut oil can increase the size of atrophic muscles. Once per day massage oil into muscles that have atrophied or diminished. Massage oil over entire body twice a week. The coconut oil is absorbed through the skin and supplies energy directly to the cells in muscles and nerves.

- Non-exhausting exercises, such as progressive resistance exercises (PRE), aerobic, speech, and respiratory. Please note that non-exhausting exercise is exercise that does not diminish the function of your body after it's done. For example, if you exercise your arms and you notice pain, weakness, or limited range of motion in them after exercising, you have exhausted your muscles and this is very dangerous. Do not exercise to the point of exhaustion.

CAUTION: Additional AKG may be necessary before and during exercise to prevent exhaustion.

Niacin, 5-hydroxytryptophan and Ubiquinol® should be taken with caution. Recent research indicates that unmetabolized niacin and CoQ10 can be toxic if located in the extracellular space between motor neurons. Up to 250 mg once daily of niacin and 50mg once daily of 5-hdryoxytryptophan, taken in the evening before sleep, is still included in Deanna's supplements to provide the precursors for NADH. Deanna still takes 400mg of Ubiquinol® three times daily. Watch www.winningthefight.org for updates!

You can find all of the supplements online. Keep in mind that not all brands are created equal! Some are higher quality and actually work better. One brand of AAKG that works well is Prima Force. WFND does not financially benefit from the purchase of Prima Force supplements. The Deana Protocol® involves many supplements. Rather than taking many different pills every day, some may prefer to simplify the therapy process by taking one substance that consists of all important supplements recommended in the Deana Protocol®. Simplesa® Nutrition has formulated a simplified version of the Deana Protocol®. A portion of the proceeds from every purchase of Simplesa®'s compound will be donated to Winning the Fight, Inc. to fund further research and improvement of the Deana Protocol®.

Additional information about what to take and not take is provided in the following chapters, but we urge you to register at www.winningthefight.org for the latest recommendations and information.

Afterword

Many conditions cause death of nerve cells, pathologically, such as ALS, Alzheimer's disease, Parkinson's disease, stroke, brain injury, glioblastoma and other neurodegenerative diseases. We now think that all of these conditions share a common denominator, insufficient energy production within the cells in order to keep the cells alive. The Deanna Protocol® program saves some of the cells at risk of cell death by supplying AKG and other substances needed to produce energy to dying cells. This has been demonstrated in our research on ALS mice.[81] The core supplements recommended in the Deanna Protocol® program are found in the body of healthy patients, and the side effects that have seen reported over the past seven years from patients around the world are mild and easily controlled.

The Weizmann Institute has conducted research in a murine model for sporadic ALS. In this model, glutamate scavengers inhibited the massive death of spinal cord neurons compared to controls.[82, 83] We hypothesize that glutamate spreads neuron death in a cascade. Dying neurons release more glutamate into the extracellular space,

---

81   http://www.researchgate.net/publication/279302050_Combined_Treatment_of_an_Amyotrophic_Lateral_Sclerosis_Rat_Model_with_Recombinant_G.

82   Ibid.

83   http://www.ncbi.nlm.nih.gov/pubmed/18423998.

which kills surrounding neurons, releasing more glutamate, killing more of the surrounding neurons, and so
on.[84, 85]

We have planned and are starting research combining
the Deanna Protocol® program with the administration
of GOT/OXA as reported by the Weizmann Institute. We
are hoping that the combination of these two modalities
prevent further neuron cell damage and spreading of the
disease to other neurons. Winning the Fight, Inc. is seeking donations to advance this research. Synthetic GOT
for treating neurological conditions is not available for
humans, and manufacturing GOT for humans requires
compliance with FDA regulatory requirements and guide-
lines. This is expensive and can be time consuming.

Conclusions About AKG and GABA

I have drawn some conclusions from having spent seven
years collecting information from individuals with ALS
from all over the world.

- <u>AKG & Muscle Twitching/Fasciculation</u>. Abnormal
  muscle contractions in neurodegenerative diseases, such as twitching and fasciculations, might
  be caused by subliminal stimuli as a result of a
  lack of energy in the cells. By taking AKG, cells are

---

84 http://www.dana.org/cerebrum/2007/protecting_the_Brain_
from_a_glutamate_storm/1v

85 http://www.alzforum.org/news/research-news/brain-imaging-
suggests-neurotransmitter-imbalance-als

provided with an alternative source of energy, and the twitching and fasciculations subside.

- GABA & Tremors/Spasticity. Muscle tremors and spasticity might be caused by a deficiency in the amount of GABA, an inhibitory neurotransmitter, compared to the amount of excitatory neurotransmitters, such as glutamate. When individuals with tremors and spasticity take GABA, tremors and spasticity subside. Based on this fact, we believe that excitotoxicity is likely caused by an imbalance between inhibitory and excitatory neurotransmitters.

Putting the Pieces Together: Glutamate, AKG, and GABA
Let's use our knowledge of chemistry in the human body and put the clinical picture together with what we know about the chemistry and see how they fit. Regarding excess extracellular glutamate, cells probably cannot metabolize and break it down as effectively because it is not inside the cell. Therefore, the body lacks the breakdown products of the Glutamate: AKG and GABA. If other pathways create AKG and GABA, these pathways are insufficient to meet the needs of PALS. When taking sufficient amounts of AKG and GABA, which varies by patient and level of activity, PALS report that the twitching, fasciculations, tremors and spasticity subside. This alone is good news for PALS, but we are hopeful that the Deanna Protocol® program can slow the progression of ALS in PALS, also. With this in mind, we are testing GOT/OXA in SOD1-G93A mice with and without the Deanna Protocol® program. We hope that

combined results of the Deanna Protocol® and GOT/OXA will further extend the life of these ALS mice, providing a strong justification for conducting clinical trials in human ALS patients. If you would like to help us, please go to www.winningthefight.org and join our cause.

APPENDIX

ALSFRS Results of Registered PALS

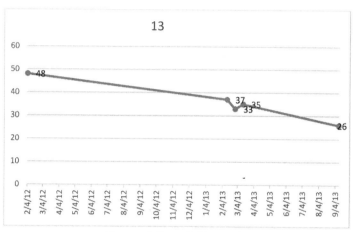

Figure 1: Loss 0.9/month

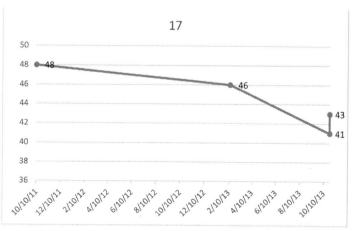

Figure 1: Loss 0.2/month

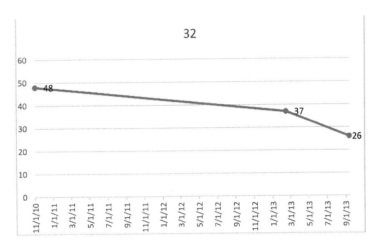

Figure 2: Loss: 0.705/month

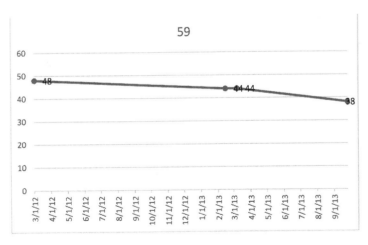

Figure 3: Loss 0.61/month

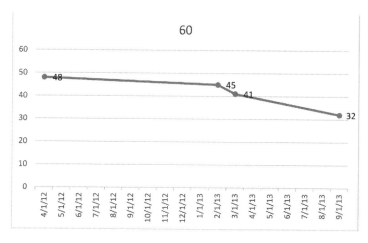

Figure 4: Loss 1.0/month

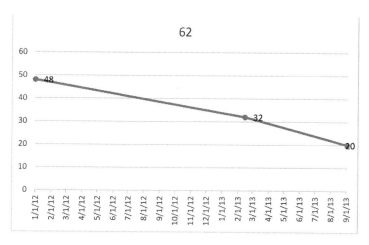

Figure 5: Loss 0.7/month

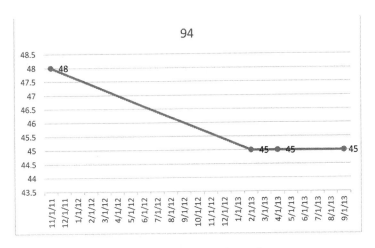

Figure 6: Loss 0.130/month

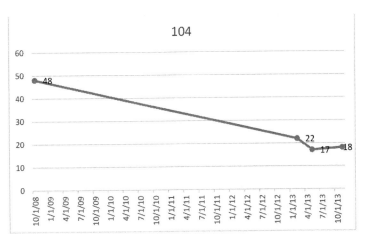

Figure 7: Loss 0.555/month

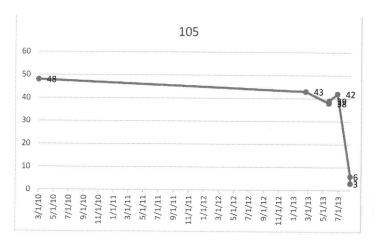

*Figure 8: Loss 0.205 (until 6/26/13) and a
39 point drop in 2 months (until 8/18/13)*

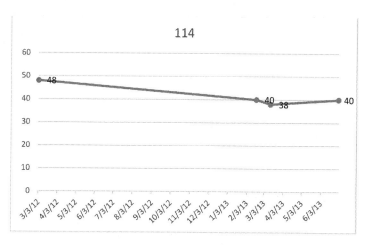

Figure 9: Loss 0.666/month

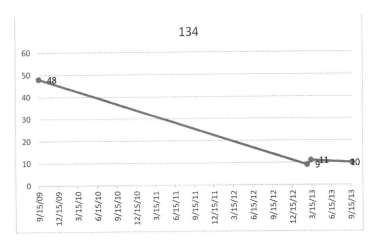

Figure 10: Loss 0.79/month

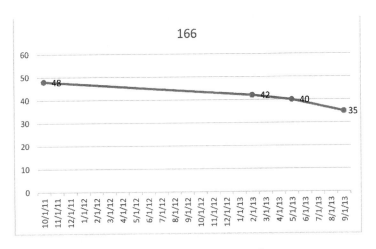

Figure 11: Loss 0.541/month

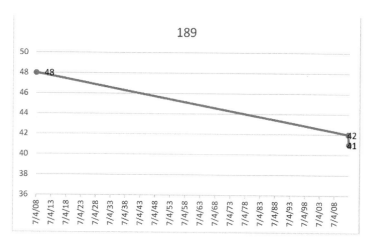

Figure 12: Loss 0.127/month

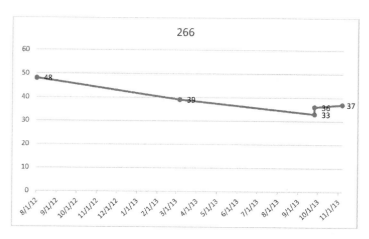

Figure 13: Loss 0.733/month

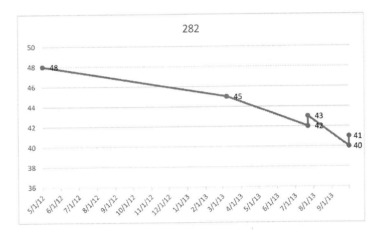

Figure 14: Loss 0.888/month

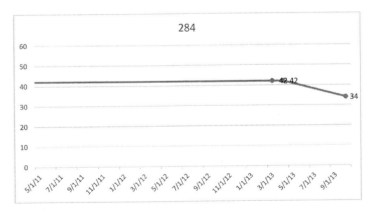

Figure 15: Loss 0.47/month

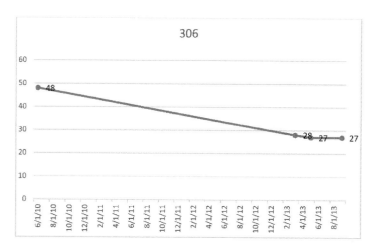

Figure 16: Loss 0.552/month

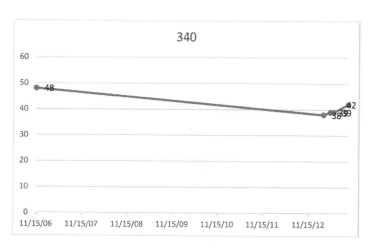

Figure 17: Loss 0.038/month

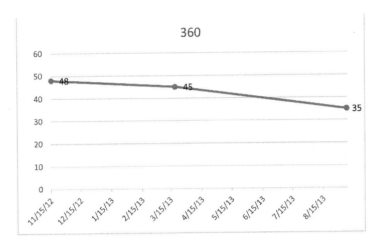

Figure 18: Loss 1.3/month

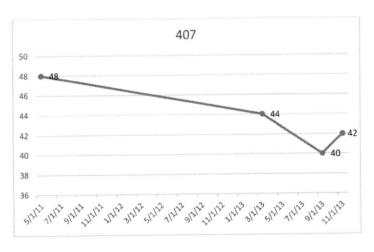

Figure 19: Loss 0.2/month

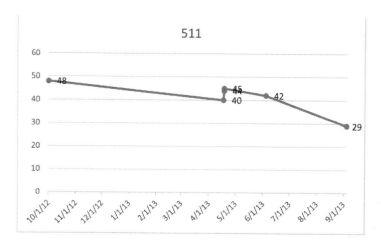

Figure 20: Loss 1.58/month

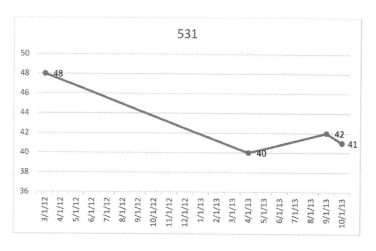

Figure 21: Loss 0.227/month

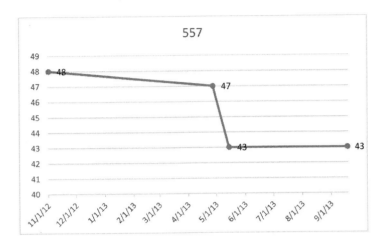

Figure 22: Loss 0.227/month

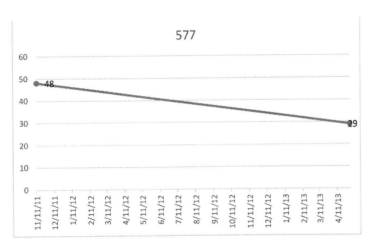

Figure 23: Loss 1.16/month

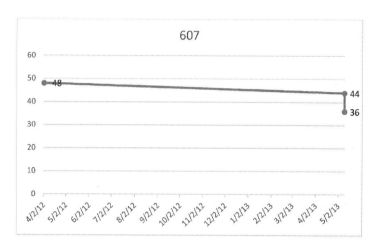

Figure 24: Loss 1.0/month

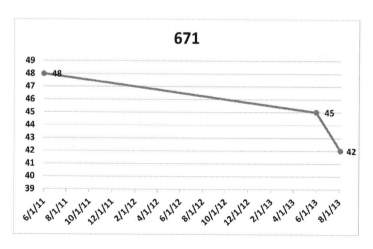

Figure 25: Loss 0.24/month

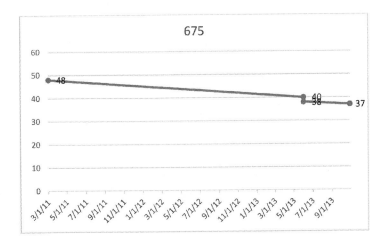

Figure 26: Loss: 0.517/month

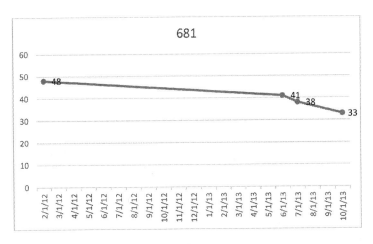

Figure 27: Loss: 0.75/month

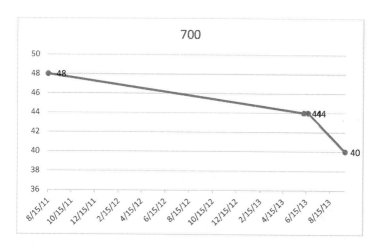

Figure 28: Loss: 0.347/month

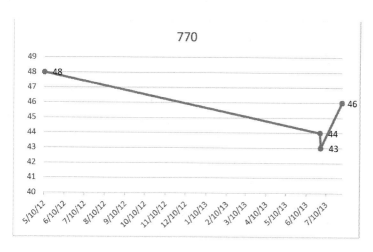

Figure 29: Loss: 0.24/month

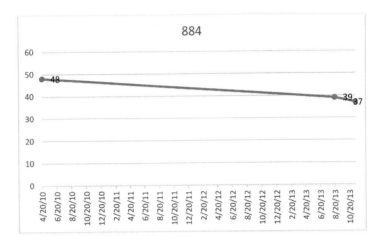

Figure 30: Loss: 0.25/month

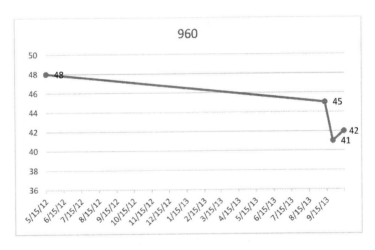

Figure 31: Loss: 0.375

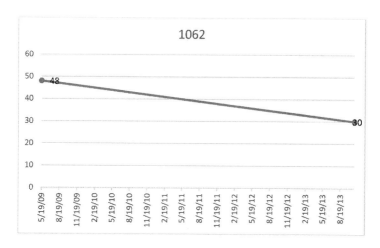

Figure 32: Loss: 0.833/month

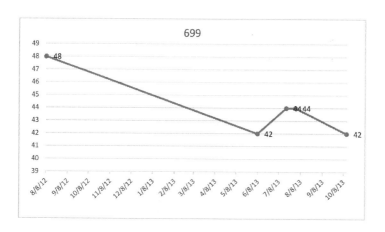

Figure 33: Loss 0.42/month

Glossary

AAKG: Arginine Alpha Ketoglutarate

ADP: Adenosine Diphosphate

AKG: Alpha Ketoglutarate

ALS: Amyotrophic Lateral Sclerosis (Lou Gehrig's disease)

ALSFRS-R: ALS Functional Rating Scale-Respiratory

Arginine: amino acid present in the body

ATP-: Adenosine Triphosphate

Baclofen®: prescription medication based on GABA

BBB: Blood Brain Barrier

chelation: the process of using organic compounds to bind metals (and remove from body).

DP: Deanna Protocol® information for use of supplements to support PALS health.

EMG: Electromyography charts electrical activity in muscle.

excitotoxicity : toxicity caused by an excess of excitatory neurotransmitters or lack of inhibitory neurotransmitters or both.

- **fasciculation:** involuntary contractions of single muscle units in muscle bundles.

GABA: Gamma Amino Butyric Acid an inhibitory neurotransmitter.

GAD: Glutamic Acid Decarboxylase enzyme that catalyzes decarboxylation of Glutamic Acid Decarboxylase.

GAD1: gene that produces enzyme GAD.

GDH: Glutamate Dehydrogenase enzyme that catalyzes a reversible oxidative de-animation of glutamate to AKG.

GLUD2: gene that encodes for GDH enzyme.

glutamate: an excitatory neurotransmitter and key compound in cellular metabolism.

GSH: Glutathione is the most effective nervous system antioxidant known to man.

GOT: Glutamate Oxaloacetate Transaminase removes glutamate from the brain by means of blood glutamate degradation. An enzyme that neutralizes glutamate by producing glutamine an amino acid.

5-hydroxtyrptophan: naturally occurring amino acid.

KB: Ketone Bodies

ketogenic diet: limits carbohydrates

Krebs cycle: energy cycle in cellular metabolism.

mitochondria: referred to as the cell's power house, providing energy to the cells.

mitochondria organelles: subunits within the mitochondria.

mitophagy: is a process for programmed mitochondria death within cells.

Motor neuron disease : diseases characterized by death of motor nerve cell.

MRI: Magnetic Resonance Imaging

Niacin: vitamin B3 or nicotinic acid.

NADH: Nicotinamide Adenine Dehydrogenase an enzyme found in all living cells.

NIH: National Institute of Health.

NO: Nitrous oxide.

oxaloacetate: is less stable than GOT substrate in the energy cycle.

PALS: patients with ALS.

phosphatidylcholine: a component of biological membranes.

PRE: Progressive Resistance Exercises.

Riluzole: a drug prescribed for ALS that extends life only a few months.

Rocephin® : antibiotic that was found to break down glutamate in a multi-institutional study funded by the NIH but failed in human clinical trials.

ROS: Reactive Oxygen Species or free radicals which do not cause as acute an inflammatory response that bacteria cause; but rather a response similar to a subacute or chronic infection that causes less swelling and hence less pain than when the inflammation is acute.

SOD1: is a gene which mutates in the familial form of ALS causing the disease.

Ubiquinol®: form of CoQ10.

WFND: Winning the Fight against Neurodegenerative Disease is a service mark of Winning the Fight, Inc., a charitable foundation established to fund research on ALS, neuro degenerative diseases and to get information to patients and caregivers.

Acknowledgments

I thank my loving husband, Don, my white knight and rock, and of course, my dad, who never gave up on finding a way to beat this awful disease. This has been a family affair from the start, and I thank my mom and sisters, Andrea and Chiara for their support. I appreciate the kindness and determination of my team of physical, speech and strength therapists, Ron Jones, Allison Zager, Brieann Yimoyines, Manisha Sharma.

The author's collectively thank all of those who have made this book possible, including Dr. Dom D'Agostino, a brave scientist, who is willing to challenge the status quo and has become like a member of our family. His research team has shown the scientific community that the Deanna Protocol® is a breakthrough for a disease where there is no cure and there was no hope. Also, we thank Walter Dykes, Dr. Erika Bradshaw, M.D., Dr. Edmund Grant, M.D., Dr. Allan Sheer, M.D., Dr. Rix Brooks, Dr. Dave Morgan, Dr. Richard Veech, Dr. Patrick Bradshaw, Dr. Csilla Aria, Dr. Randall Rush, Dr. Heather Held and all of those who have contributed their time and talent in testing the Deanna Protocol® including Angela Poff (PhD candidate), Shannon Kesl (PhD candidate), Nick Mavromates (Medical student), and Craig Goldhagen (pre-medical student).

Without the encouragement, support and advice of the board members of Winning the Fight, Inc., and the PALS that have contributed their ALSFRS scores, Paul, Steve, Warren, Andrew, Vickie and so many more, this book would not be possible, and we want to especially thank Glenn Myer, Kristine Oureilidis, Dave Thompson, Dru Movizzo, Anthony Topazi and Chris Topazi. Also, we tip our hat to Butch Machlin who informed us of the benefits of coconut oil massage.

Special thanks go to Norm Thalheimer and his wife Susan Pomeranz, who inspired the authors to believe that we could create this book. Norm conducted interviews and ghost wrote an early draft of the book. We thank Cornell Christianson for compiling a list of footnotes and for his help in writing sections of the book. We thank Mr. Alan Stephens for fighting through the original manuscript. Also, we would like to thank Mr. Jim Carlstedt for his videography on our website.

We thank the Christian Broadcasting Network for airing a story on the Deanna Protocol® at a time when we were having difficulty reaching PALS. It has helped us develop a network of PALS not only here in the U.S. but around the world.

Last but not least, I thank the publisher, paradies/inspire, llc, for never giving up on this project and for donating the time and talent of its staff to continue to make the book better.

52068330R00142

Made in the USA
Lexington, KY
15 May 2016